LIVING WELL *with* HEART FAILURE, *the Misnamed, Misunderstood Condition*

Edward K. Kasper, M.D.,
and Mary Knudson

THE JOHNS HOPKINS UNIVERSITY PRESS BALTIMORE

To the Reader

This book is not meant to substitute for medical care of people with heart failure, and treatment should not be based solely on its contents. Instead, treatment must be developed in a dialogue between the individual and his or her physician. Our book has been written to help with that dialogue.

Drug dosage. The author and publisher have made reasonable efforts to determine that the selection and dosage of drugs discussed in this text conform to the practices of the heart failure community of physicians as represented by the guidelines on heart failure published by the American College of Cardiology / American Heart Association. The medications described do not necessarily have specific approval by the U.S. Food and Drug Administration for use in heart failure or in the dosages for which they are recommended, although most of the drugs described for use in heart failure in this book have been approved by the U.S. Food and Drug Administration. In view of ongoing research, changes in governmental regulations, and the constant flow of information relating to drug therapy and drug reactions, the reader is urged to check the package insert of each drug for any change in indications and dosage and for warnings and precautions. This is particularly important when the recommended agent is a new or infrequently used drug.

Printed in the United States of America on acid-free paper
9 8 7 6 5 4 3 2 1

The Johns Hopkins University Press
2715 North Charles Street
Baltimore, Maryland 21218-4363
www.press.jhu.edu

Library of Congress Cataloging-in-Publication Data

Kasper, Edward K. (Edward Kevin), 1957–
Living well with heart failure, the misnamed, misunderstood condition / Edward K. Kasper and Mary Knudson.
p. cm.
Includes bibliographical references and index.
ISBN-13: 978-0-8018-9422-0 (hardcover : alk. paper)
ISBN-10: 0-8018-9422-0 (hardcover : alk. paper)
ISBN-13: 978-0-8018-9423-7 (pbk. : alk. paper)
ISBN-10: 0-8018-9423-9 (pbk. : alk. paper)
1. Heart failure. I. Knudson, Mary. II. Title.
RC685.C53K374 2010
616.1′29—dc22 2009024471

A catalog record for this book is available from the British Library.

All illustrations by Jacqueline Schaffer.

Special discounts are available for bulk purchases of this book. For more information, please contact Special Sales at 410-516-6936 or specialsales@press.jhu.edu.

The Johns Hopkins University Press uses environmentally friendly book materials, including recycled text paper that is composed of at least 30 percent post-consumer waste, whenever possible. All of our book papers are acid-free, and our jackets and covers are printed on paper with recycled content.

Contents

Living Well *with* Heart Failure,

the Misnamed, Misunderstood Condition

Introduction

In 2003 I (Mary) was diagnosed with heart failure. To say this was a shock is an understatement. My symptoms of fatigue and shortness of breath when walking seemed to come on suddenly. But once I had time to think beyond the emergency that took me to a hospital and a succession of cardiologists, I came to believe I had been developing for years the underlying cardiomyopathy, the heart muscle disease that caused my heart failure.

My left ventricle, the lower chamber of the left side of the heart, was enlarged; my ejection fraction, a measure of how much blood the heart pumps out in a heartbeat, was only 15–20 percent, the sign of a very weak heart. A normal ejection fraction is 55 percent or higher. My diagnosis: dilated cardiomyopathy and biventricular congestive heart failure. The dilated cardiomyopathy, which led to the diagnosis of heart failure, was labeled *idiopathic,* meaning that doctors do not know what caused it.

My experience with this disease and with the health care system made me recognize a need to alert the public to heart failure and how to take care of it. The result is this book. Eventually, we will probably learn that genetics is at least partly responsible for more cardiomyopathies than medical science is yet aware of. Other than genetics, some common and recognized causes of cardiomyopathy are coronary artery disease, heart attacks, and high blood pressure. Not so for me. An angiogram showed that my arteries were completely clear, and I have always had naturally low blood pressure. I have never had a heart attack. For half of all people who develop dilated cardiomyopathy and do not have coronary disease, the cardiomyopathy has no known cause.

I am a medical journalist accustomed to doing research about diseases, so when I got the diagnosis, I naturally began to research heart failure. I quickly came across the guidelines for treatment of heart failure recommended by a joint national panel of the American Heart Association and American College of Cardiology. I saw that I was not on two of the basic medications for heart failure, an ACE inhibitor and a beta blocker. Yet, without even trying to find out what these medicines could do for me, the third cardiologist I saw repeatedly told me that I should get a heart transplant.

Now, for someone who really needs a new heart, a heart transplant is an incredible blessing that literally provides a second chance at living. But clearly it should be a last resort. For someone like me, who had not yet experienced the most effective drug therapy, the idea of a heart transplant was unthinkable. Frightened that I could drop dead, and under the stress of seeing one doctor after another who gave me substandard treatment, I had to work to find my own path to good care.

When I found the fourth cardiologist, who immediately put me on all the medications recommended by the national guidelines, I got better. Today, I no longer have heart failure. My enlarged heart has remodeled to a normal size, and my ejection fraction is a healthy 65 percent.

I am part of an epidemic. In 2006, 5.8 million people in the United States were living with heart failure, of which 670,000 were diagnosed that year. At age 40, the risk of developing heart failure in a lifetime is 1 in 5 for men and women. As baby boomers turn 60, the number of people who learn they have heart failure will continue to grow. Heart failure is the major cause of hospitalization in people over 65. More Medicare dollars are spent on the diagnosis and treatment of this condition than on any other diagnosis.

Being informed about heart failure can help many, though not all, people avoid its perils. It is important to recognize the symptoms, which often include shortness of breath, fatigue, and swollen ankles, feet, and abdomen. If you have any of these symptoms, it is essential to get to a doctor for a diagnosis and begin taking the proper medications. The right therapy often can keep the syndrome in check and can even reverse heart damage and end the heart failure.

Heart failure is classified in stages. Doctors used to expect that most people would progress from one stage to the next until they either got a heart transplant or died. Sudden death was also a frequent occurrence.

Now many people diagnosed with heart failure will outlive it, dying of something else entirely.

Some people still do die from heart failure after having it many years. This may be the result of the heart failure's cause or severity, inadequate medical care, coexisting health problems, advanced age, or some combination. Some others die suddenly of an electrical malfunction in their heart if they are not helped in time by a defibrillator, which could have shocked their heart back to working order.

For many people, though, the journey with heart failure will be very different. Some of your most rewarding and active years at work and in your personal life may still be ahead.

To spread the truth and knowledge about heart failure, I needed a strong partner, someone trained and seasoned in treating the condition, because I wanted this book to go into detail about proper treatments for different types of heart failure. I turned to my fourth cardiologist, Edward K. Kasper, M.D., director of the cardiomyopathy and heart transplant service at Johns Hopkins Hospital when I met him, and now clinical chief of cardiology at Johns Hopkins. Ed is a leading heart failure specialist with 20 years of experience taking care of people with heart failure. He believes in evidence-based medicine and follows the national guidelines for treating the syndrome while, of course, making allowances for the needs of individual patients.

Ed and I have worked as a team in writing this book. Although all chapters reflect this collaboration, in some, one of us (or both) talks directly to readers. Ed talks to you in chapters where he can share his valuable years of experience as a doctor, such as in diagnosing heart failure, and explaining the different types of cardiomyopathies, treatments, and what it's like to be in a hospital. I speak in chapters on exercise, sudden death, and daily life with heart failure. We both talk to you in the chapter on doctor-patient relationships. Every chapter in the book is the product of our joint research, our experience, asking each other tough questions, and collaborating on the writing and revising. This book is a team effort of a medical journalist and an internationally known heart failure specialist, a woman diagnosed with heart failure and her doctor. Nutrition is an important part of living well with the condition, and for the nutrition chapter we turned to Samantha (Sam) Heller, Ed's childhood friend from third grade, who is now a well-known nutritionist. Through this book, we want you to empower yourself with knowledge about heart failure—how to treat it, what questions to ask your doctors, what potential problems to avoid, and how to take charge of your life and your heart failure.

One thing that *I* learned was that having asthma need not prevent you from receiving the best therapy for heart failure. My second cardiologist wondered aloud to me why I was not on a beta blocker and suggested that it may be because I have asthma. He, too, did not put me on a beta blocker, which is proven through clinical trials to help relieve heart failure, restore a heart to its normal size, and extend lives. Many doctors are reluctant to prescribe beta blockers for people with asthma, but doctors need to become informed about the differences among these medications. Many people with asthma can take a beta blocker such as metoprolol succinate, which blocks primarily the beta one receptor. Except if used at high doses, this type does not interfere with asthma medication, which works by using the beta two receptor. Two other common beta blockers used in heart failure block both receptors, and people with severe asthma who sometimes need to rely on a rescue inhaler should avoid those beta blockers.

As you read this book, you can learn more about whether you are getting the best treatment for your heart failure. If you are not, ask why and get an answer you understand and agree with, get your treatment changed, or move on to another doctor.

Life is choices. I can only wonder where I would be today and how I would be feeling if I had been a passive patient and let myself get placed on a heart transplant waiting list.

I, along with you who have heart failure, are the new face of heart failure in the twenty-first century. Many, many of us will not proceed to death from heart failure. We will not proceed to transplantation. We will just proceed.

Mary Knudson

Caring for people with heart failure has been a central focus of my adult life. I (Ed) have seen some people struggle with this syndrome and others flourish. Many factors go into who will do well and who will not with heart failure. A well-informed patient is my best partner. He takes the time to understand his disease and what he can do for himself. She understands what her medications, diet, and exercise can do for her heart failure and follows the path we agree is right for her. Questions are always welcome, because they demonstrate an interest in what is happening. I believe this is critical in becoming one of the people likely to do well.

This book is a place to start. Learn as much as you can about heart failure. Participate in your care. Knowledge and participation will serve you well. We wrote this book to help you. Although I cannot be your doctor, and neither can this book, Mary and I hope it sets you on the right path. We hope you get well as Mary has gotten well. Good luck and happy researching.

Edward Kasper, M.D.

Part I

The CAUSES *and* DIAGNOSIS *of* HEART FAILURE

1

What Is This Thing Called Heart Failure?

You notice that you get out of breath easier and more often than you used to. In a weekend game of tennis, the chief competition becomes the game itself. Walking up a flight of stairs at work instead of taking the elevator is no longer an option. Carrying groceries into the house or mowing the lawn requires stopping to catch your breath. Soon, taking a shower becomes a chore, and the side of the tub you have to step over seems to keep getting higher. Maneuvering your foot into that first pant leg and pulling it up while staying balanced is a challenge, and after dressing, you sit down because you're breathing heavily.

"Boy," you think, "am I out of shape!" But if you also feel tired frequently and notice swelling in your ankles, legs, or abdomen, or watch the bathroom scales inch upward when you haven't added a pint of Häagen-Dazs to your daily diet, please listen to your body talking. And take that body to a doctor. The reasons you've thought of—being out of shape, putting on weight along with years, having trouble with asthma or allergies—may not be the right reasons.

You may have heart failure, formerly known as congestive heart failure. Not everyone with this condition experiences all the same symptoms, and your symptoms may have started suddenly or they may have come on gradually. Fatigue, breathlessness, swelling, weight gain—any or all of these may be symptoms of heart failure. You will see that many, but not all, symptoms are due to "congestion." The preferred name these days is *heart failure,* rather than *congestive heart failure,* for just this reason.

Heart failure is a medical name given to a heart that has begun struggling to do its job and no longer meets the body's needs during normal activity. Several different diseases or abnormalities in the heart and major blood vessels can bring on heart failure. It's worth repeating this important concept: heart failure is not a disease; rather, it is a syndrome, a condition of the heart that can be caused by a disease or other abnormality of the heart or blood vessels.

Many definitions of heart failure say that it means a weakened heart. That's a tempting definition, but it is true in only about half the people with the syndrome—those whose heart has become large and stretched. A person can have heart failure and not have a weakened heart. The second most prominent type of heart failure occurs when the left ventricle becomes stiff, and as a result, the heart doesn't fill well with blood. Or a person can have a completely normal heart muscle and yet develop heart failure if a heart valve becomes narrowed and blocks blood flow, or if an abnormal connection between arteries and veins forces the heart to do extra work to pump blood, which then returns to the heart prematurely. There are other causes of the condition, too.

Because heart failure may mean an enlarged and weakened heart, or a heart that pumps strongly but fills poorly, or a normal heart with abnormal connecting blood vessels, or a narrowed heart valve, creating a short definition gets tricky. We can say that *in heart failure, the heart and cardiovascular system are unable to provide the blood and oxygen that the body needs*.

If it is not treated, heart failure will progress, and shortness of breath may eventually occur even when the person is resting. In advanced heart failure, a person may awaken suddenly at night and sit upright, gasping for breath. This can occur anytime while lying down (it just so happens that most of us try to sleep at night). Some people with heart failure feel a need to sleep with their head elevated on two or more pillows in order to breathe freely, or even to sleep sitting up in a chair. Coughing can be an early sign of difficulty breathing. A cough that is worse lying down and better sitting up may be a manifestation of heart failure. As you can imagine, all this shortness of breath disturbs sleep, leaving a person markedly fatigued. It can even precipitate sleep apnea, which causes a person to periodically stop breathing while sleeping and then restart with a loud snort or snore. In addition to driving a partner from the bedroom, sleep apnea causes daytime sleepiness, falling asleep at inappropriate times, irregular heartbeats, and worsening heart failure.

CAUSES OF HEART FAILURE

Coronary artery disease, which we discuss in much more detail in chapter 2, is the major cause of heart attacks and of heart failure in the United States. With improved treatment, more people are surviving heart attacks (the medical term is *myocardial infarction*). But many people who survive are then at risk for developing heart failure, because a portion of the heart muscle dies during a heart attack. Once heart muscle dies, it can no longer participate in the crucial contracting, pumping action that is the sole function of the heart. If the area that died is large, the heart's ability to pump is weakened. Think of a baseball team trying to win a game with its entire infield missing. This form of muscle damage, known as *ischemic cardiomyopathy*, leads to heart failure.

Ischemic cardiomyopathy is one of several types of cardiomyopathies with various causes. Cardiomyopathy is a disease of the heart muscle itself. People who have coronary artery disease and people who do not can develop cardiomyopathy. For half of all people who get it, there is no known reason; doctors have labeled this idiopathic cardiomyopathy. While some cardiomyopathies weaken the heart's ability to pump, others stiffen the heart, making it unable to fill properly with blood. We discuss the different cardiomyopathies in chapter 3.

Any condition or disease that impairs the ability of the heart to function as a pump at normal pressures and volumes can cause heart failure (see "What Can Go Wrong," later in this chapter, as well as chapters 2 and 3). Why is it so important for your heart to pump at a normal strength and send a normal amount of blood through your body at a normal pressure? And why does a heart that no longer pumps strongly enough cause shortness of breath and fatigue? An understanding begins with some basic human anatomy and physiology.

HOW THE HEART WORKS

We need oxygen to create energy to do the things we do. In the process of using energy, our bodies make carbon dioxide, which we need to constantly exhale and replace with oxygen to live. The heart and lungs and a maze of arteries, veins, and capillaries make this happen. The heart is a simple, elegantly constructed muscular pump that is hollow because blood must flow through it. The heart continually pumps blood

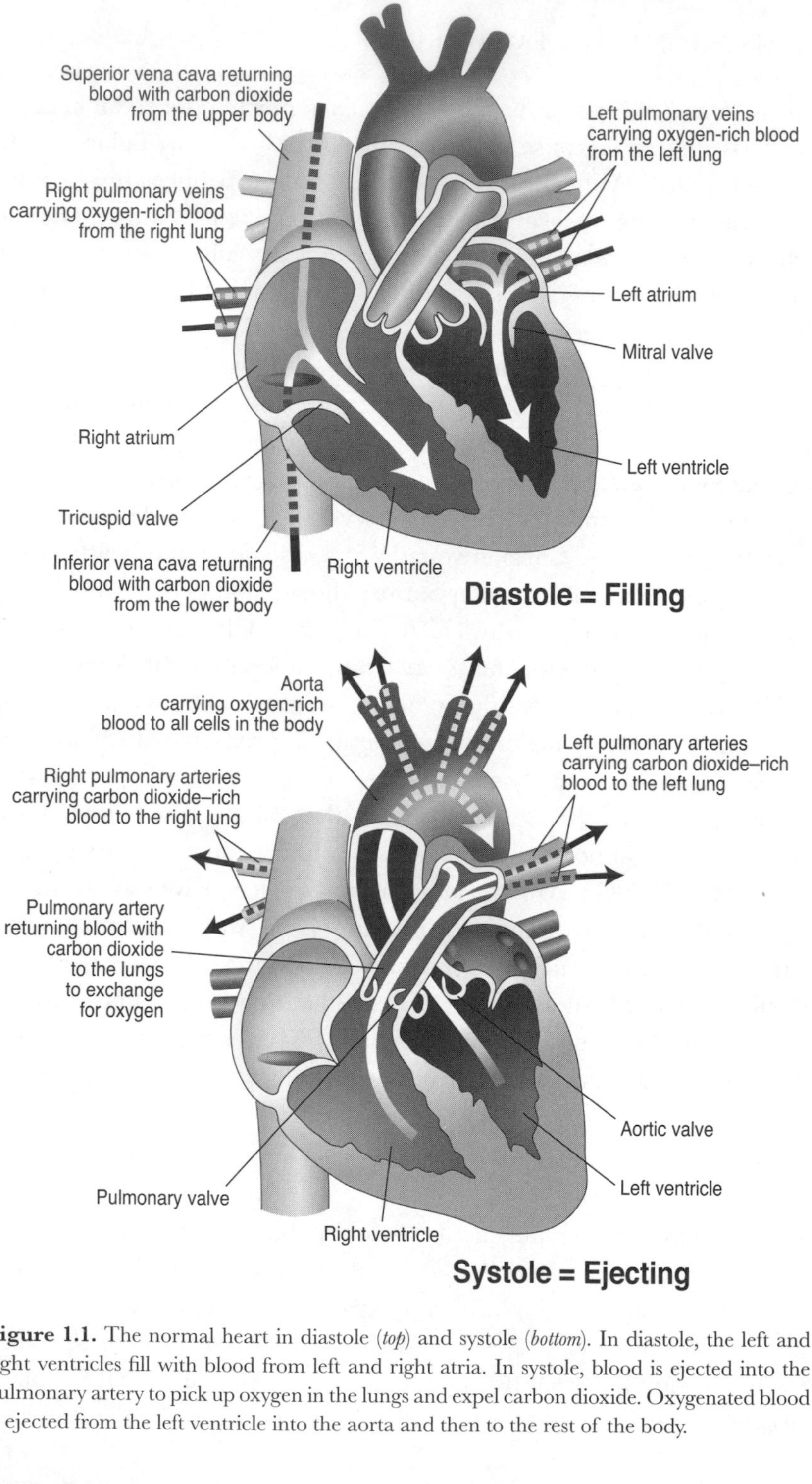

Figure 1.1. The normal heart in diastole (*top*) and systole (*bottom*). In diastole, the left and right ventricles fill with blood from left and right atria. In systole, blood is ejected into the pulmonary artery to pick up oxygen in the lungs and expel carbon dioxide. Oxygenated blood is ejected from the left ventricle into the aorta and then to the rest of the body.

throughout the body. The blood picks up oxygen from the lungs and carries the oxygen to all parts of the body, then picks up carbon dioxide and returns it to the lungs, which exhale it. The blood completes this trip around the body in about a minute.

The Blood's Round Trip

The heart is the body's Atlanta airport, the hub through which all blood traffic passes on its round trip, when returning carbon dioxide from the body to the lungs and when carrying oxygen from the lungs back to the body. The heart has four chambers and four valves. Blood flow from one chamber to another is controlled by the valves—gates that open and close to keep blood moving in only one direction (figure 1.1). The four valves are made of tough, flexible tissue that is nearly transparent and does not contain muscle. While the four valves have the same purpose of regulating blood traffic, they have different shapes. The walls of the heart are all muscle and can contract like any other muscle.

Transporting carbon dioxide, blood returns from the body in veins and enters the first of two right chambers of the heart, the *right atrium.* Blood flowing into the right atrium needs a way to move on to the next chamber of the heart, so the first valve (the *tricuspid valve*) opens its three tightly closed sections outward like petals of a flower, creating a passageway for the blood to flow into the next chamber, the *right ventricle.* Then the ventricle contracts, causing the petals of the tricuspid valve to close. The closed valve prevents the blood from flowing back into the right atrium. Now the second gate, the *pulmonary valve*, opens, and the blood rushes through it into the large pulmonary artery, beginning its trip to the lungs. From the pulmonary artery, blood feeds into progressively smaller arteries until it gets to the lung's capillaries, which are so small that red blood cells can literally move only in single file, like bumper-to-bumper cars that must pass through a toll booth before entering a tunnel. Instead of giving up two dollars and passing through, the cells give up carbon dioxide, which we quickly exhale, and pick up oxygen to take to the body.

To get back out to the body, the blood must return to the body's hub, where it will go through the two chambers that make up the left side of the heart. And so, from the lung capillaries, blood travels through progressively bigger veins until it gets to the *left atrium* of the heart. Now a gate must open to let the blood into the *left ventricle.* The third gate, the *mitral valve,* looks like the mouth of the heart, with lips that open and close. Blood crosses through the open mouth into the left ventricle. When that ventricle contracts, the mouth closes, and blood leaves the heart by way of the fourth gate, the *aortic valve,* to get to the aorta. Then the aortic valve closes to prevent the blood from running backward into the heart. (The aortic valve is the valve that most often becomes abnormal in older people.)

To recap, the blood that traveled through the body returned to the right side of the heart to move to the lungs, where it disposed of its carbon dioxide and picked up oxygen. Then the blood returned to the left side of the heart and moved into the aorta, ready to move out and refuel the body with oxygen. From the *aorta,* the body's largest artery, blood travels through progressively smaller arteries until it gets to capillaries throughout the body. In the narrow enclosures of the capillaries, the red blood cells again line up in single file, and this time they exchange oxygen for carbon dioxide. A minute is up. A round trip completed. And the next round trip immediately begins. What a journey! It's a wonder we don't feel the blood coursing through our bodies, and hear the raucous swooshing noises it makes; but since our blood makes this round trip about 1,440 times a day, aren't we glad we don't!

You can see that in fact the heart is two pumps that work in a coordinated sequence of perfectly regimented events. The right heart, which is the right atrium and the right ventricle, pumps blood containing carbon dioxide to the lungs, where it is exhaled, and then the blood picks up oxygen. The left heart—the left atrium and left ventricle—pumps blood carrying oxygen to all parts of the body.

The Pump and the Electrical System

The heart generates pressure like any other pump. In this case, the pressure moves blood through the circulatory system. The major pumping, or pressure-generating, chambers of the heart are the two ventricles. To generate pressure, the muscular ventricles squeeze, or contract. When the pressure in the ventricles is greater than the pressure in the arteries, the heart ejects blood to the lungs and the rest of the body. This part of the cardiac cycle represents the highest pressure in the arteries and is called *systole.* After ejecting blood, the ventricles must again fill up with blood. This part of the cardiac cycle, when the pressure in the arteries is lowest because the heart is at rest, is called *diastole.*

The ventricles fill with blood from the heart's receiving chambers, the left and right atria. Again, when the pressure in the atria is greater than the pressure in the ventricles, blood will flow down this pressure gradient into the ventricles like water going downhill. *Each chamber of the heart has a volume of blood and a pressure at which it operates best.*

Your blood pressure has two components, systolic and diastolic, which is how blood pressure is measured. A blood pressure of 110 over 70 means that in systole (highest pressure in the arteries) your blood pressure is 110 mmHg (millimeters of mercury), and in diastole (lowest pressure) it is 70 mmHg. Too high a pressure causes blood vessels to rupture, while too low a pressure means that tissues don't get enough blood.

This is a good place to remind you of the connection between pressure and volume and heart failure. Any condition that impairs the heart's ability to fill with blood or to eject blood at the pressures and volumes at which the heart normally operates causes heart failure. The pump can fail either because it doesn't fill up properly or because it doesn't contract with adequate force. In either case, the output of that pump—the volume of blood leaving the heart every minute—will be inadequate to nourish the body. When a person is resting, the demands placed on the diminished heart are minimal, and the volume of blood leaving the heart may be adequate. With exertion, however, the heart is called on to increase blood flow. With a normal heart, this is not a problem. But with heart failure, the heart is not able to meet this demand, and symptoms develop. If it is not treated, heart failure worsens because the heart becomes less and less able to pump out enough blood, and the amount of exertion needed to cause symptoms becomes smaller and smaller until, ultimately, symptoms occur at rest.

To coordinate all its precise contractions and valve openings and closings, the heart has an electrical system. Nerves run from the brain to the heart to control the rate at which the heart contracts. We know, though, that the heart doesn't require this connection to the brain to function effectively because in a heart transplant operation, in which a person's damaged heart is removed and replaced with a new heart, these nerves from brain to heart are severed and do not usually grow back. Yet the new heart usually works well.

The heart can get along without the electrical signals from the brain because it has an intrinsic electrical system to coordinate its own contraction. The electrical signal begins high up in the right atrium, spreads to both atria, and then moves down to a traffic control station, the *atrioventricular node* (or *AV node*), in the middle of the heart, about halfway between the atria and the ventricles. This traffic delay station slows down the speed of the electrical impulses, allowing time for the atria to contract and fill the ventricles before the ventricles contract. If both atria and ventricles contracted at the same time, no blood flow would occur because there would be no difference in pressure to move the blood. From the traffic station, the electrical signal is spread to the ventricles by the *right bundle branch* and the *left bundle branch,* special heart muscle fibers made to conduct electricity. When both these bundles of fiber are working correctly, they allow the ventricles to contract at the same time. (See figure 1.2.)

Just like every other muscle and organ, the heart needs oxygen. Blood that goes through the inside chambers doesn't deliver oxygen to the

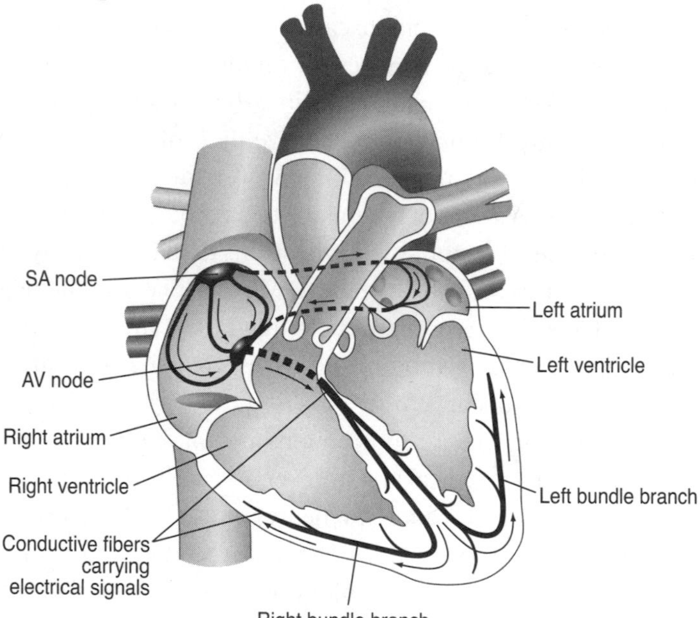

Figure 1.2. The normal electrical system of the heart. The pacemaker of the heart, the sinoatrial (SA) node, located in the right atrium, fires an electrical charge that spreads through both the left and right atria to the atrioventricular (AV) node. Here the pulse slows, allowing time for the atria to contract before the ventricles. From the AV node, the electrical wave spreads through special conductive fibers called the right and left bundle branch to activate the right and left ventricles.

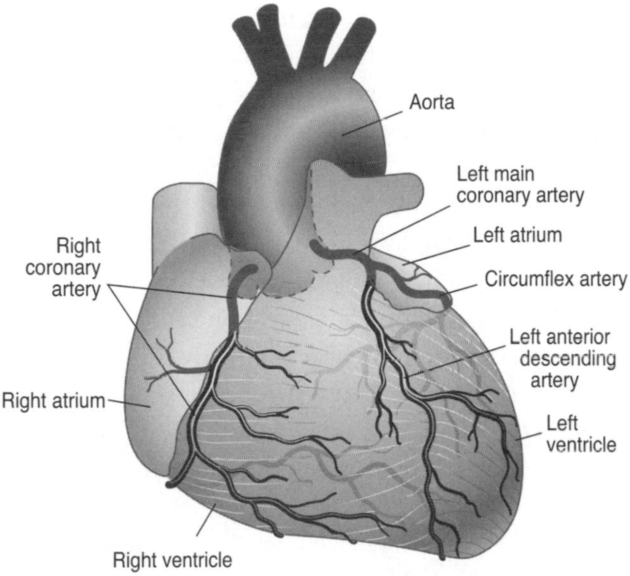

Figure 1.3. Blood supply for heart muscle. The heart has its own system of arteries, capillaries, and veins. The coronary arteries bring blood to the heart muscle itself. There are two major coronary arteries, the right and the left main coronary artery. The left main coronary artery splits into the left anterior descending coronary artery, which runs down the front of the heart, and the circumflex coronary artery, which runs around the left side of the heart. The right coronary artery runs around the right side of the heart and often will supply the backside of the heart as well (not depicted).

heart. To get this oxygen, the heart has its own system of arteries, capillaries, and veins just like any other organ. There are two main coronary arteries, the left and the right. The left very quickly divides into the *left anterior descending*, which runs down the front of the heart, and the *circumflex*, which runs around the left side of the heart. The right coronary artery snakes around the right side of the heart. (See figure 1.3.) The heart operates within a sturdy sac called the *pericardium*, which separates the heart from the lungs.

WHAT CAN GO WRONG

A problem with virtually any part of the heart can cause heart failure. Here are examples:

- Cholesterol deposits can pile up inside coronary arteries, over time building to an eruption that stops blood passage. Without blood, heart muscle located beyond the blockage dies during a heart attack. Dead heart muscle cannot contract, leaving too much work for the rest of the heart to do.
- Cardiomyopathies cause problems with the muscle of the heart. Causes of cardiomyopathy are explained in chapter 3.
- Valves may leak, allowing blood to travel backwards; or they may fail to open completely, making ejection of blood difficult.
- The electrical system may cause the heart to beat too slowly or too quickly or out of sync. Many people with heart failure have *left bundle branch block* in which the special fibers in the left bundle branch slow the electrical current. When this happens, the electrical signal takes longer to get past the left bundle (located on the left side of the left ventricle) than it does going directly through the right bundle (located on the right side of the left ventricle). As a result, the right and left sides of the left ventricle do not beat in sync.
- The pericardium surrounding the heart may shrink, wrapping so tightly around the heart that it restricts the heart's ability to fill with blood.
- The circulation itself may be abnormal. There might be an abnormal connection between an artery and a vein, for instance, a connection that bypasses the capillaries and may bring excessive amounts of blood back to the heart.
- Other causes of heart failure are listed in chapter 4 (see especially the boxes in that chapter).

WHAT CAUSES THE SYMPTOMS OF HEART FAILURE?

When something goes wrong with the heart, why does a person get short of breath and fatigued?

Whatever the cause of the person's heart failure, as the heart delivers less blood, the body reacts with a stress response. Here is one theory about why that happens: The brain and kidneys sense a diminished blood supply and react as though the person has been wounded and is experiencing blood loss. That's because people haven't inherited genetic information for coping with heart failure. By the time people are at an age where heart failure most often occurs—fifties, sixties, seventies—

they have already had their children, so those who survive heart failure aren't selectively able to pass their body's know-how on to the next generation. But mammals, including humans, *have* inherited genes from the fittest who survived blood loss from wounds or other causes, so we do have mechanisms for coping with a lowered blood supply. Our bodies don't recognize the difference between an inefficient heart pump—the medical condition we call heart failure—and loss of blood due to an emergency caused (centuries ago) by an animal attack or (today) by a car accident or a shooting. So the body responds to what it thinks is an emergency. That's the theory about why the body responds as it does to heart failure.

What then takes place is known. During an emergency, most of us have experienced a rush of adrenaline that provides an extra boost of energy. When our brain signals a fight-or-flight response, we can feel our heart beat faster. In heart failure, the sympathetic nervous system secretes *norepinephrine,* a hormone very similar to adrenaline, and the kidneys discharge *renin,* a hormone that initiates release of a string of other hormones to create *angiotensin II.* These powerful hormones, norepinephrine and angiotensin II, cause the heart to beat more forcefully, pumping out more blood. That would be useful if a person were truly wounded and needed a short-term boost to the heart to keep more blood flowing before getting to a hospital, where the bleeding would be stopped. Once the bleeding stopped, the outpouring of hormones would also stop.

But on a long-term basis in people who have heart failure (and are not wounded), this continuous hormonal drenching becomes harmful to the heart. It's like having the gas pedal in your car stuck to the floor and not being able to ease off the flow of gas. The flood of hormones acts like a stimulant that tries to turn your heart into a souped-up race car engine. But nobody's heart was built to be a race car engine other than for a short-term emergency or an athletic event. And, obviously, a heart that was already struggling to do its job and falling behind can't be forced along at a high rate for an extended period. It just struggles and, like a sputtering, chugging car engine, could conk out. (See figure 1.4.)

As part of the body's response to stress, we hold on to sodium and fluid, and our urine becomes concentrated and dark yellow. We get thirsty and drink more. This is a great response to blood loss because it helps to restore normal plasma volume, the liquid part of the blood. For heart failure, though, fluid retention leads to trouble. Unexplained

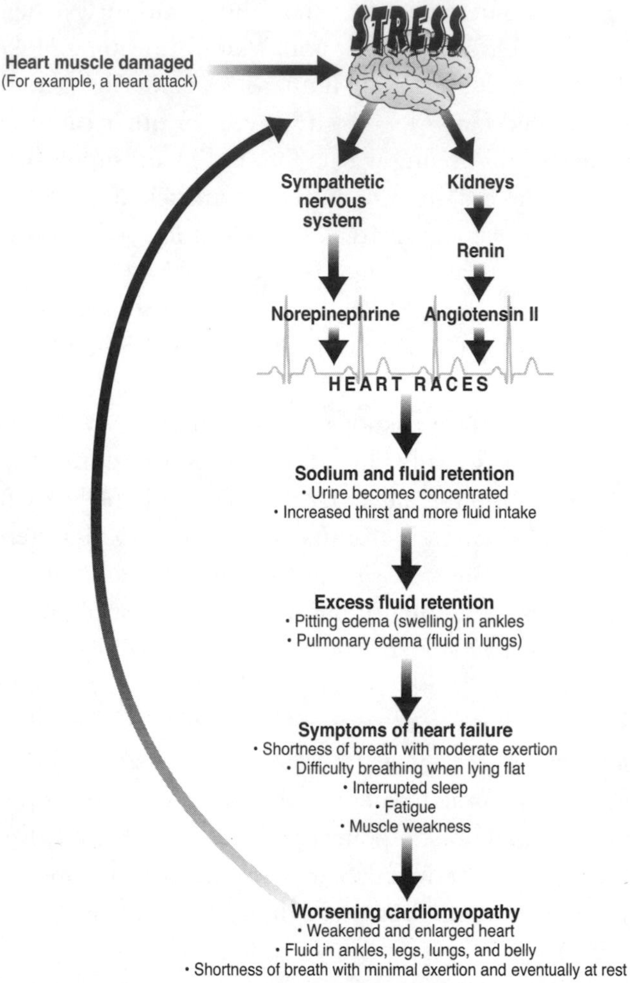

Figure 1.4. Vicious cycle of neurohormonal activation. An initial insult such as a heart attack damages the heart, which leads to the release of various neurohormones, such as norepinephrine from the adrenal glands and renin from the kidneys. This is how the body handles a stress response. These neurohormones are initially beneficial but in the long term become harmful. They increase the symptoms of heart failure and worsen the function of the heart, which leads to the release of more neurohormones in a vicious cycle.

weight gain may be a tip-off that your body is retaining fluid when you have no need for extra fluid, so you become relatively waterlogged. The excess fluid is found in many places. Gravity tends to cause fluid to pool in lower areas—usually those closest to the ground, like our feet and ankles. A sign of heart failure is *pitting edema* of the ankles. Pitting means that if you press your thumb into your ankle, the imprint is left behind for five seconds or longer as a pit, or indention. Edema means swelling with fluid, and it can occur in the lungs as well. Normally, the lungs are like a moist sponge filled with many air pockets. Lungs filled with fluid are like a wet sponge right out of a bucket of water, so those air pockets are filled with fluid. Obviously, a person with such fluid-filled lungs will strain to breathe.

To understand what makes it hard to breathe when lying flat or why a person might wake up at night gasping for breath and quickly sit up, we need to understand a bit about what goes wrong with the pressures and volumes inside the heart in heart failure. Remember, each chamber of the heart has a pressure and a volume of blood at which the heart is most efficient as a pump. When a weakened left ventricle fails to contract adequately, fluid and the pressure that fluid causes build up in the left ventricle. This increase in pressure and volume will be passed backwards along the blood's pipeline of blood vessels, heart chambers, and lungs. The increase in pressure is passed back to the left atrium and eventually to the capillaries in the lungs. Here the increased pressure causes fluid, which is the clear portion of blood, to leak from the bloodstream through the capillary walls and into the lungs themselves, causing fluid buildup in the lungs. Ultimately, this increased pressure can also be passed back to the right ventricle, the right atrium, and eventually the capillaries in the body, leading to fluid retention in the ankles, legs, and even belly.

When we lie down and put our feet up on the bed, we basically give ourselves a transfusion. When we sit and stand during the day, blood tends to pool in the veins of our legs and belly due to the effects of gravity. Putting our feet up allows this pooled blood to move back toward the heart, where it may overwhelm the heart's pumping abilities, leading to fluid leakage into the lungs, causing us to strain to breathe. Coughing is an early manifestation of wet lungs, and waking up at night needing to sit up immediately to get a breath is an extreme manifestation of finding it difficult to breathe.

This shortness of breath leads to deconditioning and is a factor in atrophy of skeletal muscles, and the extra work of breathing leads to fatigue of the muscles involved in breathing. All of these harmful processes make us unable to do the things we would like to do.

The fatigue of heart failure can be due to interrupted sleep caused by difficulties breathing while lying down. It can also be due directly to diminished flow of oxygen-rich blood to the body. If the heart cannot provide active muscles with the blood and oxygen they need, the muscles will be limited in what they can do. Because fatigue is a very common symptom and is usually not due to heart failure, you or your doctor may, unfortunately, explain your fatigue by saying it's caused by a lack of conditioning, overwork, or getting older. Misinterpreting the causes of fatigue can delay a diagnosis of heart failure.

Chest *pain* is not really a manifestation of heart failure. It is more commonly a symptom of coronary artery disease, which we describe in chapter 2. People with heart failure may get a *pressure feeling* in the chest even if they do not have coronary artery disease. This is because the higher pressure in the lungs caused by heart failure is sensed as a tightening, or constricting, sensation in the chest.

WHAT ARE THE STAGES OF HEART FAILURE?

The New York Heart Association classifies four stages of heart failure. People with Class I heart failure have no symptoms, meaning they are no more short of breath than people without heart failure. People with Class II heart failure have shortness of breath with moderate exertion, such as walking upstairs while carrying a bag of groceries. In Class III, people get short of breath with minimal exertion, such as walking a short distance on level ground. Class IV patients have shortness of breath and fatigue at rest.

Another classification comes from the American College of Cardiology (ACC) in association with the American Heart Association (AHA). In this classification, heart failure is divided into four stages labeled A, B, C, and D. In Stage A, risk factors for heart failure such as high blood pressure or diabetes mellitus exist, but no physical problems have developed in the heart or connecting blood vessels. In Stage B, tests reveal that physical heart problems have developed, but the person has not yet experienced symptoms of heart failure. An example is someone with a weak left ventricle who is not yet short of breath. In Stage C, a person has symptoms of heart failure in addition to physical heart problems. And in Stage D, a person has symptoms so severe that standard therapy no longer provides relief. The ACC /AHA classification system is a useful scheme for doctors, who can tailor therapy to the degree of symptoms as well as to the presence of underlying heart disease.

The diseases that lead to heart failure are usually progressive, meaning that without treatment, people progress through the four stages. But with the improved treatments now available, this no longer has to be the case, and often it is not.

2

Coronary Artery Disease

The Major Cause of Heart Failure

Coronary artery disease is the major cause of heart failure because it blocks arteries, and open coronary arteries are necessary to bring essential oxygen to the heart muscle. Cholesterol is often painted as the enemy of arteries, but the enemy of arteries is not cholesterol. It is excess cholesterol.

Cholesterol is a fatty, waxy substance that our body makes to use in cell membranes, tissues, digestive juices, and both male and female hormones. It is so essential that the liver and most of our cells manufacture all the cholesterol we need. The excess cholesterol we don't need comes from food—trans fats, saturated fats, and cholesterol itself. Eating trans fats and saturated fats is actually more harmful than eating cholesterol because these types of fats cause the liver to increase its cholesterol production. This raises your levels more than eating cholesterol itself does.

Cholesterol moves in our blood from one part of the body to another. Because it is a waxy substance that would quickly clog up a blood vessel, our body encases it and other fats in a protein, transforming it into a lipoprotein that can travel through the bloodstream.

Which brings us to the names of the two types of cholesterol, one destructive and one helpful. Low density lipoprotein (LDL) is dubbed the bad cholesterol. These lipoprotein particles have a lower density because they contain more fat and less protein. Any LDL the body doesn't need—any excess LDL—heads for arteries and lodges in artery walls. High density lipoprotein (HDL) has more protein and less fat. HDL is called the good cholesterol because it sweeps up LDL and whisks it to the liver, where it is turned into useful bile acids or removed from the body. This is how HDL does no damage and, in fact, helps us. Eating trans fats increases LDL levels and reduces HDL levels, so it is very important to avoid food containing trans fats. They cause so many health problems that some parts of the country have passed laws prohibiting restaurants from using them in cooking.

Maintaining the right balance of cholesterol is key. When your cholesterol is checked in a blood test, more important than the total cholesterol number is the breakdown: How much of that total number is LDL, and how much is HDL? If you have a high HDL number and a low LDL number, you probably don't need to worry, even if your total cholesterol number is above normal. How low your LDL level should be depends on whether you are at risk of developing coronary artery disease or already have it. If you have had a heart attack, your doctor will want you to lower your LDL cholesterol level. If you do not have known coronary artery disease, your target LDL level will depend on whether you have risk factors for the disease, such as diabetes and tobacco use. The more risk factors you have, the lower you should get your LDL. Risk-based LDL levels for coronary artery disease are shown in table 2.1. These risks are discussed in detail at the end of this chapter.

Why avoid excess LDL cholesterol? Because it can build up in an artery wall. Inflammation occurs, and the body summons immune cells and grows a *fibrous cap* over the mound of cholesterol and immune cells. Frequently, these fibrous caps will break open. This rupture of a cholesterol deposit is a disaster because it can cause blood to clot at the rupture

Table 2.1. Recommended LDL Levels for People at High, Moderate, and Low Risk of Coronary Artery Disease

Risk level	*Recommended LDL level*
High (previous heart attack or known coronary artery disease)	<70 mg/dl
Moderate (diabetes mellitus, tobacco use, family history of heart attacks, metabolic syndrome, high total cholesterol, high blood pressure)	<100 mg/dl
Low (no presence of coronary artery disease or major risk factors)	<130 mg/dl

Source: National Heart, Lung and Blood Institute, National Institutes of Health, *Detection, Evaluation, and Treatment of High Blood Cholesterol in Adults (Adult Treatment Panel III)*, 2002, updated in 2004.

site. The hardened cholesterol deposits, known as plaque, take years, often decades, to form. But the rupture and blood clot happen in minutes or even seconds, and they are a life-threatening emergency because the clot can completely block the opening of the artery.

If blood cannot get past the clot, the heart muscle beyond the blockage dies from lack of oxygen. The death of part of the heart is a heart attack (myocardial infarction). If just a small section of the heart is affected, the person had a small heart attack. If a large part of the heart is affected, the person had a massive heart attack. How much of the heart is affected depends in part on where the clot occurs; there is less damage if the clot forms in a branch of an artery, and more damage if it forms in a major artery. Once part of the heart muscle dies, the rest of the heart that is still healthy must work harder to make up for the lost area. This extra work can lead the heart to become weak, enlarged, and in heart failure.

Coronary artery disease is very common, and it is the most common cause of a weak heart muscle. In 2006, 17.6 million people in the United States had coronary artery disease, and 425,425 people died from it, according to the "Heart Disease and Stroke Statistics—2010 Update," published by the American Heart Association. The coronary artery disease death rate dropped by 36.4 percent from 1996 to 2006, but this disease, and the heart attacks it causes, remains the single leading cause of death in America today.

Atherosclerotic deposits in arteries can occur throughout the body, causing *atherosclerosis,* also known as hardening of the arteries; when these plaques occur in coronary arteries, this is coronary artery disease, also called coronary heart disease or, more simply, coronary disease. Decades before we deposit fat in our coronary arteries, however, we begin to develop atherosclerosis in our abdominal aorta. The aorta is the major artery that runs from the heart down to about the belly button, where it splits into branches that continue down the legs. The portion of the aorta in our abdomen seems particularly prone to deposits of fat, which begin in many of us in our twenties and thirties. Note, however, that even if you are genetically prone to developing belly fat, you are not necessarily more susceptible to developing fat in your abdominal aorta. The two processes are not connected.

THE VIEW INSIDE AN ARTERY

To understand the process of fat and cholesterol collecting in our arteries, we need to know how the normal artery works. More than just a pipe, a coronary artery is made of three structures, each with a distinct purpose (figure 2.1). Innermost is the *intima*, a single layer of endothelial cells and surrounding tissue whose true purpose was for a long time unknown. These cells were first considered simple paving stones lining the inside of the blood vessel to keep blood from leaking out. We now know they are truly remarkable cells. Far from being inert paving stones, these critical cells are actually small factories, constantly producing a variety of ingredients necessary to keep blood liquid.

The function of the intima is crucial, because blood that is not touching endothelial cells will clot. That's as it should be. The process of clotting helps us avoid death by bleeding when we're injured, for example. But *where* in our bodies blood clots is all important. If a clot forms inside an artery or vein, blood can't flow past the clot, and cells and other tissues downstream of the clot will die. A clot in a coronary artery leading to our heart can cause a heart attack and possibly death. In the *carotid artery* that runs through our neck and into the brain, a clot can cause a stroke.

Deeper into the wall of the artery, separated from the endothelial cells by a membrane, is the structure called the *media*. The arterial media resembles stretch pants or a girdle made of smooth muscle cells interlaced with a stretchy material called *elastin*. The give and take of the media allows the artery to get larger (dilate) when increased blood flow is needed and get smaller (contract) when less blood flow is needed.

The outpost of the arterial wall is the third structure, the *adventitia* (pronounced ad-ven-ti-sha), a loose connective tissue containing nerves and small blood vessels. The nerves signal smooth muscle cells to contract, constricting the blood vessel and decreasing blood flow. The tiny blood vessels bring blood to the walls of the artery. After a big meal, for instance, blood is shunted to the gut to aid in digestion and away from the arms and legs, so arteries in the gut dilate, and arteries in the arms and legs constrict.

The lives of blood vessels are even more complicated than we have described, however, because the walls of different blood vessels are

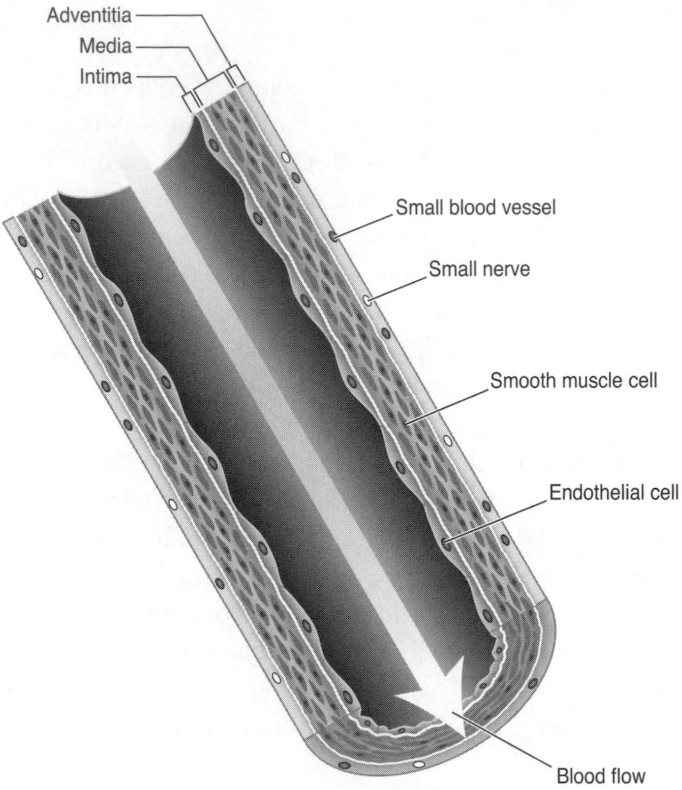

Figure 2.1. Structures of a normal coronary artery. The three parts of a normal coronary artery are the intima, media, and adventitia. The intima is composed of endothelial cells. The media is largely made up of smooth muscle cells and elastin. The adventitia consists of loose connective tissue, small blood vessels, and nerves.

built more from one type of material than from another. Large arteries have more smooth muscle cells and elastin. Smaller arteries have fewer smooth muscle cells and less elastin. Veins have the three-component structure but differing amounts of smooth muscle cells and elastin.

HOW DOES A PLAQUE DEVELOP?

All arteries, regardless of their exact makeup, are subject to the fatty buildup of atherosclerosis. We know that this cholesterol buildup is more likely to occur in certain locations in certain arteries, but we don't know why. Perhaps it has to do with blood flow itself, because atherosclerosis tends to occur at branch points of arteries, where blood must flow into multiple smaller arteries. Blood flow at these branches becomes turbulent, and the rough, choppy blood flow may increase the likelihood of fat and cholesterol deposits. This turbulence injures some of the endothelial cells. Tobacco also injures endothelial cells, whether through smoking or through passive exposure to tobacco smoke. These assaults provide openings for the fat and cholesterol deposits to move across or between the endothelial cells and into the inner lining of the artery. White blood cells, the part of blood that is largely responsible for fighting infection, begin to accumulate alongside the fatty deposits in the arteries. Normally, white blood cells do not cross into the lining of an artery, so this accumulation represents an abnormal response, called inflammation.

Once white blood cells are in the artery's wall, a specific type of white blood cell, called a *macrophage,* begins to swallow the fatty lipoprotein particles, and the macrophages become "foam cells," so named because they look foamy under a microscope. Foam cells produce various stimuli that draw other cells involved in inflammation into the inner wall of the artery. Smooth muscle cells, which are normally part of the midsection of the artery wall, are drawn into the innermost layer of the artery—where they should not be. Foam cells begin to die, leaving their collection of fats and cholesterol behind in a soupy mix of foam cells, smooth muscle cells, fats, and cholesterol.

And that's how a plaque develops. A mature atherosclerotic plaque has a fat-and-cholesterol-rich core surrounded by a fibrous cap of scar-like tissue that is covered with an outer layer of endothelial cells. Initially, the plaque grows outward, away from the inside of the artery, expanding the outside of the artery. The plaque encroaches on the inner, hollow area of the artery, where blood flow occurs only once the plaque exceeds 40 percent of the normal opening of the artery. As plaque continues to build up, the hollow area of the artery becomes progressively smaller, until eventually blood flow is compromised. We can see why coronary artery disease is described as "clogged pipes." The *process* of clogging the artery is very complex and occurs over several decades. (See figure 2.2.)

ANGINA: A SYMPTOM OF ARTERIAL DISTRESS

When the passageway is narrowed by about 60 percent, blood flow becomes limited in times of increased demand, such as when the person is exercising or experiencing intense emotions: anger, grief, fear, or sometimes even happiness. The limited flow causes *angina*, which can be experienced as chest pain or as an oppressive pressure in the middle of the

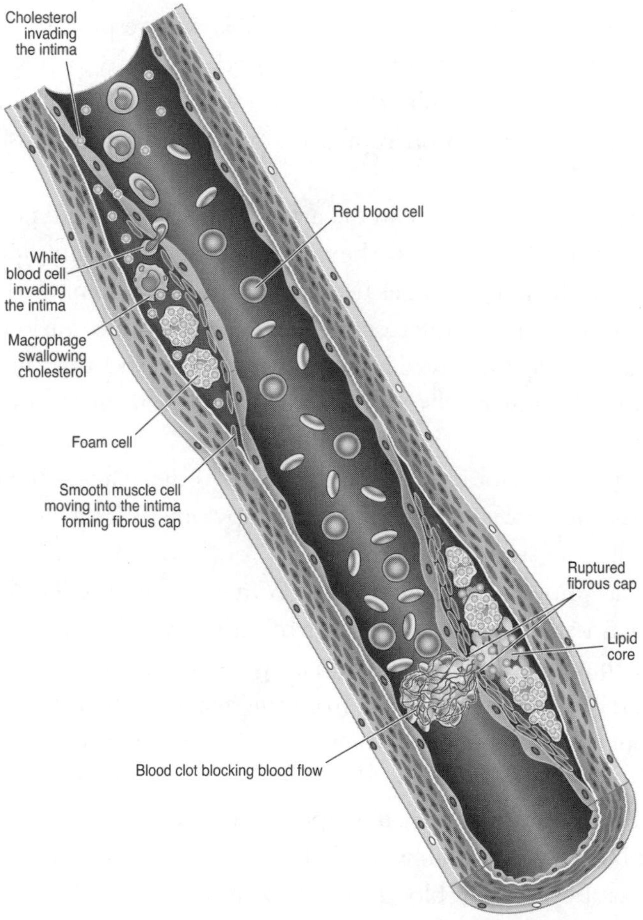

Figure 2.2. The development of atherosclerosis, leading to plaque rupture and a heart attack. The upper part of this figure shows the development of a cholesterol plaque, including the presence of foam cells, white blood cells, and smooth muscle cells. The lower end of the figure shows rupture of a cholesterol plaque, leading to blood clot formation and blockage of the artery.

chest. Angina often involves discomfort in the shoulders, jaw, or neck and travels down the left arm more commonly than the right. It is expressed in many forms. Some people feel it only in their shoulders; others describe it as more like a weight in the chest than as pain or pressure. The bottom line is that *any sensation above the waist and below the nose that comes on with exertion and goes away with rest could be angina* and should be discussed with your doctor. This type of angina is called *stable angina,* and treatment may include medications such as beta blockers to decrease demand for coronary blood flow.

A more serious kind of angina, called *unstable angina,* occurs when a person is at rest. It shares many features with and is a major predictor of a heart attack. Doctors use the term *acute coronary syndrome,* or ACS, to refer to both a heart attack and unstable angina. Unstable angina, like a heart attack, is an emergency that must be treated immediately by medications such as heparin or another anticoagulant (blood thinner).

Angina and unstable angina used to be commonly treated by inserting a stent to keep the artery open or by *coronary artery bypass grafting* (CABG), commonly known as bypass surgery. These procedures are designed to push the blockage out of the way and keep it out of the way. Coronary bypass surgery is open-heart surgery in which detours are created around the blockages using arteries removed from the inside of the chest wall or veins removed from the legs. Cardiologists are reconsidering using stents for stable angina, however, because a large clinical trial called COURAGE, reported in 2007, found that stenting for stable angina or stable coronary artery disease did not prevent heart attacks or deaths. This major study conducted at fifty medical centers in the United States and Canada found that aggressive medical therapy (a combination of different medications and a strict diet) worked just as well. However, if medications fail, stenting or CABG is often recommended to control angina symptoms.

The critical event for both a heart attack and unstable angina is nearly always rupture of the fibrous cap of the atherosclerotic plaque. Once the cap ruptures, the bloodstream is exposed to the contents of the lipid core, a thick liquid that is an extremely good catalyst for clotting. And so a 50 percent narrowing by plaque that took years to build up can suddenly become a complete blockage within a matter of seconds. The blockage is the result of a plaque rupturing and forming a blood clot, not of the plaque itself. If the blockage is only partial and some blood flow remains, unstable angina occurs. If the blockage is complete, a heart attack occurs because, once blood flow stops, the heart muscle beyond the blockage begins to die.

A completely occluded coronary artery is an emergency that requires immediate coronary stenting or clot-busting drugs in an effort to open the clogged artery. Better treatment has helped lower the death rate from coronary disease, but speed is of the essence—speed in recognizing that something is wrong; speed in getting to the hospital emergency room; speed in recognizing the heart attack; and speed in beginning treatment—because with every minute that passes, heart muscle is dying. If a balloon must be inserted to open an artery, doctors have less than 90 minutes from the time the patient arrives at the hospital.

If the heart attack goes unrecognized or untreated and damage is done, cardiac muscle will not grow back. It is replaced by scar tissue that does not participate in the crucial contracting function of the heart. This leaves the heart weak and sets up the possibility of heart failure.

RISK FACTORS FOR CORONARY ARTERY DISEASE

Of course, better than any treatment is *prevention* of coronary disease. Primary risk factors for the disease are smoking, high blood pressure, high cholesterol, family history, inactivity, obesity, dietary factors, mental stress, and depression. Also at risk are people who have metabolic syndrome. Let's examine each of these risk factors in turn.

Cigarette Smoking

Cigarette smoking is the single most important risk factor under our control, and quitting is the single most important thing we can do to prevent coronary disease.

Tobacco injures endothelial cells, creating openings for cholesterol to lodge in an artery wall. In one study, quitting smoking reduced death due to coronary disease by 36 percent compared with those who continued to smoke. The reward for quitting is a prompt and significant decrease in risk for coronary disease. Smoking reduction, except as a waystation to complete cessation, has only a minimal effect on decreasing risk. Even secondhand exposure to tobacco smoke from cigarettes, pipe smoking, and cigar smoking increases heart disease risk, although not as great a risk as posed by directly inhaled cigarette smoke. Sadly, cigarette smoking is becoming a bigger problem in adolescents, young adults, and women in the United States as well as in people who live in the developing world.

High Blood Pressure

High blood pressure (also called *hypertension*) is the silent assassin. It damages endothelial cells and causes other changes in the blood vessel wall and in the heart, leading to deposits of cholesterol and causing heart attacks, strokes, aneurysms, kidney failure, and heart failure. Almost one-third of people who have high blood pressure are undiagnosed, and of those diagnosed, only one-fourth are effectively treated. This bleak situation is particularly common in the African American population. High blood pressure is defined as having an elevated systolic blood pressure reading (top number) or an elevated diastolic blood pressure reading (bottom number). A normal blood pressure is 120/80. High blood pressure means either the systolic is greater than 140 or the diastolic is greater than 90. Readings between normal and high blood pressure are considered *prehypertension*, and whether treatment is needed requires careful consideration. The majority of people with high blood pressure will require two or more medications to achieve good blood pressure control. You may need to work with your doctor over a period of months to find both the right dose and the combination of medicines that work for you.

High Cholesterol

There is clearly a link between high cholesterol levels in the blood and coronary disease. People with high LDL blood serum cholesterol levels (*hyperlipidemia*) are at increased risk of death from coronary disease by developing a plaque that ruptures and causes a heart attack. However, your LDL score alone does not predict a heart attack. Excess LDL is just the first step in a plaque buildup. No one can tell you if you will actually experience a plaque rupture and formation of a blood clot. Heart-healthy diet and drug treatment regimens decrease the risk of death. We begin developing our cholesterol levels early in life, so that is the best time to begin building a healthy lifestyle with exercise and a diet that excludes trans fats and is low in saturated fats and cholesterol.

Genetics

Coronary disease can run in families as a result of a genetic predisposition. Most of the genetic disorders that lead to coronary disease, however, have not been identified. Of those that are known, some are mutations in the receptor that normally clears LDL cholesterol from the bloodstream. The mutation prevents this clearing. While HDL helps pick up cholesterol deposited by LDL in the tissues, including artery walls, the LDL receptor clears LDL from the bloodstream itself. Since we cannot select our biological parents, inherited abnormalities can only be watched for and worked with. They cannot be prevented. Reductions in other risk factors may help slow or prevent the coronary artery disease process in someone who is genetically predisposed to developing the disease.

Inactivity and Obesity

Inactivity and obesity are closely tied together as coronary disease risk factors. The heart-protective effects of exercise include a decrease not only in weight but also in blood pressure, diabetes (or risk of diabetes), and hyperlipidemia (excess fat and cholesterol). There is a strong relationship between level of daily exercise or activity and death from coronary disease. We discuss exercise in chapter 13.

Nutrition

Lower risk for coronary disease is generally associated with a diet high in fruits and vegetables, whole grains, legumes, fish and fish oil, poultry, and some lean meat. A diet low in saturated fats, trans-fatty acids, and sugar is associated with a decrease in coronary disease risk. Modest consumption of alcohol—one or two glasses per day—is also associated with decreased coronary disease risk. If your heart failure was caused by excessive drinking, however, it is better not to drink alcohol at all. Nutrition is the topic of chapter 12.

Mental Stress and Depression

Mental stress and depression both strongly predict coronary disease. Other personality characteristics, such as increased anger and hostility, also appear to be related to the disease. Scientific studies are in agreement with people who believe their heart attack was due to stress. In addition, natural disasters such as earthquakes and floods appear to be associated with an increase in coronary death among those who survive the disaster.

Metabolic Syndrome

Metabolic syndrome is a medical disorder that increases the risk of diabetes and heart disease. The syndrome is diagnosed in a person with a combination of any three of the following: elevated blood sugar (>100 mg/dl), abdominal obesity, high blood pressure, increased serum triglycerides, or low HDL cholesterol levels. Having diabetes alone is associated with an increased risk of coronary disease, but the risk increases greatly in someone with metabolic syndrome.

Other Risk Factors

A risk factor more recently linked to coronary disease is increased presence of inflammation. Inflammation can be measured through blood tests for *C-reactive protein* (CRP), but the test is not specific for inflammation of the arteries. No evidence to date shows that lowering CRP decreases the risk of developing coronary disease. Research into this issue is under way.

Other risk factors being explored are elevations of *homocysteine* and *lipoprotein(a)*. Homocysteine is an amino acid important for growth. It is a product of the breakdown of another amino acid, methionine, which is found in fish. A rare genetic defect that prevents a person from breaking down homocysteine results in high levels of the amino acid and coronary disease. The normal level of homocysteine in the blood (fasting) is 5–15 umol/L. Homocysteine is broken down by a process that depends on folate and other B vitamins. Though folate and other B vitamin supplements lower homocysteine levels, it has not been shown that taking these supplements lowers the risk of coronary disease or stroke.

Lipoprotein(a), which is a modified form of LDL, seems to have a special ability to cause plaques. Unless the levels are very high, however, it appears to be associated with only a minor increase in risk for coronary disease, and there are few accepted treatments to lower lipoprotein(a) levels. Because of this, thc level is seldom measured except in labs with a special interest in measuring it for research purposes.

Coronary disease is very common, but the risk of developing it is decreased in a body that allows the heart and blood vessels to do their best job. If you smoke, you must stop. Make that a priority in your life now. Get your blood pressure and cholesterol levels tested, and if they are high, work with your doctor and a nutritionist to lower them.

Obesity is becoming an epidemic in our country. You can take control of what you eat and how much you move. You can set up an exercise routine at home or at a gym. Consider working with a personal or group trainer to help you stay motivated and involved. (See chapters 12 and 13 for tips and ideas.)

A predilection for coronary disease is something we inherit, but it is also something we control through our actions. We cannot change our parents, but we can exercise; eat whole grains, fruits, and vegetables; avoid trans fats altogether; eat little saturated fat; and avoid tobacco smoke.

3

Cardiomyopathy

A Leading Cause of Heart Failure

Cardiomyopathy is a disease of the heart muscle itself and is a leading cause of heart failure. There are different types of cardiomyopathy and still a good bit of mystery about them. The symptoms people notice and the signs doctors see vary widely. Response to treatment and prognosis is usually not predictable. Some people with cardiomyopathy are severely ill, while others do not even know they have it.

Causes vary for the different kinds, and half of all people with dilated cardiomyopathy have an idiopathic process, which means doctors don't know what caused it. A cardiomyopathy can lead to heart failure in various ways. The two most frequent are when the heart grows too large and weak and can't eject enough blood to supply the body's needs, and when the heart gets so stiff it can't fill properly with blood. There are four types of cardiomyopathy: *dilated*, *hypertrophic*, *restrictive* (figure 3.1), and a rare inherited form called *arrhythmogenic right ventricular dysplasia*. Let's look at each type.

DILATED CARDIOMYOPATHY

I (Ed) remember seeing Jonathan for the first time like it was yesterday. He was short of breath just sitting in my office. He couldn't walk without becoming extremely short of breath. His shoes did not fit because his feet and ankles were*

**Names of patients in this chapter and the brother of one have been changed to protect their privacy.*

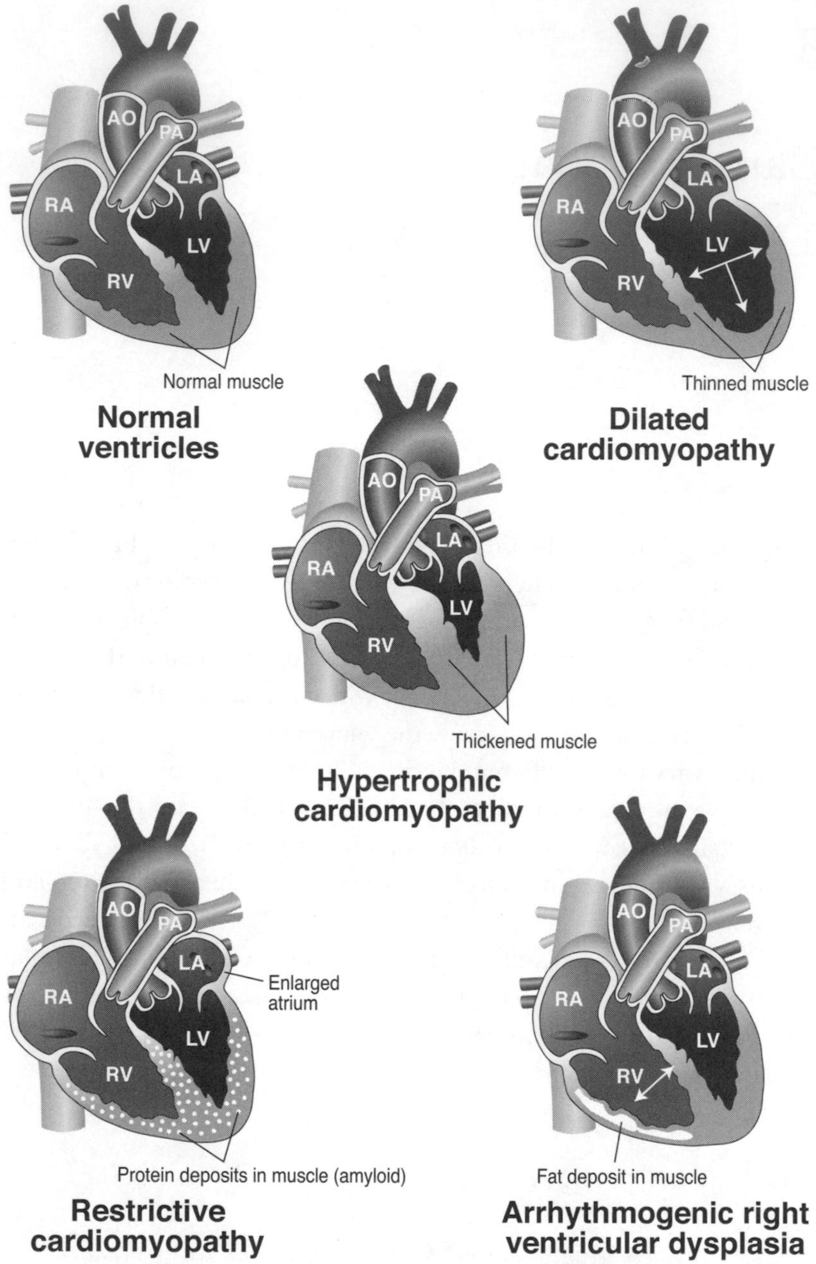

Figure 3.1. Classification of cardiomyopathies. The four types of cardiomyopathy include dilated, hypertrophic, restrictive, and arrhythmogenic right ventricular dysplasia. In dilated cardiomyopathy, the left ventricle is enlarged with decreased ability to contract. In hypertrophic cardiomyopathy, the left or right ventricular wall thickens. Restrictive cardiomyopathy is characterized by stiff but not particularly thick ventricular walls and large atria. In arrhythmogenic right ventricular dysplasia, the right ventricular wall is largely replaced by fat.

swollen, and he told me he had just bought a new belt and new pants because he had retained so much abdominal fluid that his old ones no longer fit. Further, he told me he had difficulty sleeping nights because he woke up gasping for air. I spent just enough time with Jonathan to learn about his symptoms and give him a quick examination before I sent him right to the hospital for therapy.

Jonathan had extreme symptoms of heart failure caused by dilated cardiomyopathy, the most common type. It draws its name from the enlargement (*dilation*) of either the left ventricle or the right ventricle, two of the four chambers of the heart. Bigger is definitely not better. The enlarged heart is less powerful, not more powerful. And a weaker heart is less able to squeeze blood out to the rest of the body.

Doctors can estimate the squeezing power of the heart with a formula called the *ejection fraction*. This formula, expressed as a percentage, is the amount of blood pumped out of the left ventricle with each heartbeat divided by the amount of blood in the left ventricle just before it begins to squeeze. We measure the ejection fraction by watching the heart's pumping action in "real time" in an echocardiogram, a test that uses sound waves to visualize the heart. The ejection fraction for a normal heart is not 100 percent. It is 55 percent to 65 percent. If our hearts operated at rest with an ejection fraction of 100 percent, we would have no reserve to get up and do anything that required exertion—not even walk. A reading much below 50 percent is considered abnormal and indicates a diagnosis of dilated cardiomyopathy. Jonathan's ejection fraction was 20 percent.

People with dilated cardiomyopathy are the people with heart failure who most often have noticeable symptoms. We don't know why this is so. On the other hand, as many as half of the people with dilated cardiomyopathy have no symptoms at all. They have yet to develop heart failure. If their cardiomyopathy is not treated, however, they will develop heart failure. These people find out they have dilated cardiomyopathy only when a routine electrocardiogram done for some other medical reason reveals abnormalities, after which they typically will have an echocardiogram, which pinpoints the heart's trouble. In people with cardiomyopathy, sudden death is not uncommon. It usually occurs because the heart develops a very fast heartbeat, an arrhythmia called *ventricular tachycardia*, and then goes into *ventricular fibrillation*, an electrical convulsion that makes the heart shake uncontrollably instead of beating, rendering it useless. (We discuss abnormal heart rhythms and sudden death in chapters 6 and 7.)

When I first saw him, Jonathan had never experienced chest pain and had not suffered any fainting spells, which can result from a very rapid heartbeat. I was asked to see him by his community cardiologist, who had performed a cardiac catheterization procedure to find out why Jonathan was short of breath. The catheterization showed that Jonathan did not have coronary artery disease but that the pressures inside his heart were abnormally elevated. His echocardiogram revealed a dilated left ventricle and the low ejection fraction of only 20 percent.

In the hospital, Jonathan responded well to standard medical therapy, which at that time was intravenous diuretics, digoxin, and an angiotensin-converting enzyme inhibitor. But I noticed that he found it difficult to get out of a chair, and he had a peculiar walk. I asked a neurologist who specialized in neuromuscular diseases to see him, and lo and behold, the neurologist diagnosed a congenital muscle abnormality. Jonathan had a type of muscular dystrophy that can weaken not only the muscles of the arms and legs but also the heart muscle.

After he left the hospital, Jonathan began taking a beta blocker in addition to his other medications, and he did well for several years until he began to have progressive symptoms of heart failure once again. This time, despite medications, it became more and more difficult to keep him out of heart failure, and he was admitted to the hospital repeatedly. During one admission, his heart went into ventricular tachycardia and he fainted. Since the fainting was a warning that he might experience sudden death, we put an implantable cardioverter defibrillator (ICD) in his chest, with electrical leads attached to his heart that would provide an electric shock if his heart again went into a potentially deadly wild beating pattern. The shock would save his life by righting the heart's rhythm so that the heart would once again function as a pump. Eventually Jonathan underwent heart transplantation and has done very well. He has no symptoms of heart failure and has returned to work full time at an office job.

There are many causes of dilated cardiomyopathy, including, most commonly, coronary artery disease, high blood pressure, and genetics. The most common cause is coronary artery disease (discussed in chapter 2). People with a history of heart attacks may have a significantly damaged heart with a low ejection fraction. High blood pressure may also weaken the left ventricle and cause a dilated cardiomyopathy. It is thought that the higher the blood pressure and the longer it goes untreated, the greater the chance of developing a dilated cardiomyopathy. Dilated cardiomyopathy can run in families, and a number of genes have been identified that predispose a person to it. If no cause for the person's disease can be found, family members should be screened for dilated cardiomyopathy with an electrocardiogram and an echocardiogram. If the disease does run in the family, affected members can receive early treatment. This is very important, and it is worth repeating: *a person who has no symptoms but whose tests show physical signs of dilated cardiomyopathy will very likely develop heart failure unless treated.*

Some people with cardiomyopathy are told they had "a viral infection" of their heart. Many viruses can infect the heart, but only a few cause any problems. Why these viruses cause problems is a matter of speculation. Some researchers believe that the virus and the heart muscle cells share certain components of their cell walls. In an effort to rid the body of the virus, the body causes an immune reaction, which also targets the heart because of these shared cell wall components. After the virus is long gone, the immune reaction persists, causing heart damage. We call this *myocarditis*, inflammation of the heart muscle, which may lead to dilated cardiomyopathy. It is not clear how commonly this occurs. The only real way to make a diagnosis of myocarditis is with a heart biopsy. We can test the blood for inflammation, but these tests cannot determine if the inflammation is in the heart or somewhere else. Most patients who have been told they had a viral infection of their heart have not had a heart biopsy. It would be more honest to say, "We don't know what caused the dilated cardiomyopathy."

Another type of dilated cardiomyopathy occurs in women without a history of heart disease who are either in their last month of pregnancy or in the first five months or so after delivery. This is *peripartum cardiomyopathy*, which, luckily, often resolves spontaneously or with medical therapy. However, it is always a particularly emotional issue because the woman is so young and has at least one very young child.

Other causes of dilated cardiomyopathy include various medications, alcohol, cocaine, and endocrine diseases such as thyroid problems. I often tell patients that the list of causes, if typed single spaced, would be six feet long. This is an exaggeration but not too far from the truth. A few of the causes of dilated cardiomyopathy have specific treatments, but most causes do not. Therefore, an exhaustive look for the cause is usually not needed or useful. When doctors cannot find a reason for the dilated cardiomyopathy, it is usually considered an idiopathic case. This is a frequent finding.

Regardless of the cause, if left ventricular function is impaired and is not treated, a vicious cycle is set in motion: left ventricular remodeling occurs, in which the heart grows bigger and even less able to beat efficiently. As compensation for low blood pressure and poor output of blood from the heart, the body reacts with a variety of responses designed to bring blood pressure and blood flow back to normal. As animals, we are designed to survive blood loss. The body evokes a stress response that works for blood loss but doesn't work for dilated cardiomyopathy. This stress response includes the outpouring of several hormones, including norepinephrine and angiotensin II. In the short term, this works. In the long term, this response increases the work of the heart, which causes it to stretch and become more dysfunctional.

A low ejection fraction will not inevitably get worse. Sometimes the ejection will increase on its own. Medications may increase it and reverse the remodeling process. The lower the ejection fraction, the worse the cardiomyopathy, and the greater the risk of death. In more than 15 years of seeing patients with heart failure, however, I have learned that the ejection fraction does not necessarily predict a person's symptoms or ability to exercise. Some people with a low ejection fraction don't get out of breath during normal exertion like walking up a short flight of stairs, while others with a moderate to nearly normal ejection fraction do. Though progress is made every year in understanding heart failure, there are still mysteries left to be solved.

Because dilated cardiomyopathy involves problems when the heart is actively squeezing to eject blood (the systole period), heart failure caused by this type of cardiomyopathy is called *systolic heart failure.* Two other types of cardiomyopathy, hypertrophic and restrictive, cause *nonsystolic heart failure,* because they affect the heart when it is filling with blood, not ejecting it.

HYPERTROPHIC CARDIOMYOPATHY

Amanda was a young woman with a problem. We knew what it was because her whole family had the same problem. It was initially picked up when her older brother, Ty, died suddenly while playing baseball in high school. Autopsy showed that he had hypertrophic cardiomyopathy, which is an enlargement of the walls of the left, right, or both ventricles. Because this condition can run in families, all of Ty's family members had an echocardiogram and an electrocardiogram. From these tests we learned that Ty's father and his sister, Amanda, both had the disorder.

Both of Amanda's tests were markedly abnormal. This is not always true in hypertrophic cardiomyopathy. Even if you inherit one of the genes responsible for the condition, you may not develop a severe case of the disorder. Amanda had few symptoms. She did not then, and more than 10 years later still does not, have heart failure. When I took her medical history, I learned that she had already experienced some worrisome lightheadedness spells. Because of this symptom, her test results, and her brother's sudden death, I recommended that she get an ICD. Eleven years later, the device had shocked her heart one time, and it had probably saved her life. She has done well, works full time, and is a mother. Her father had multiple shocks from his defibrillator. He eventually needed a heart transplant, which is rare in hypertrophic cardiomyopathy, and since then has continued to do well.

If dilated cardiomyopathy is the seventy-pound weakling, then hypertrophic cardiomyopathy is the muscle-bound weightlifter. The enlargement may involve the entire left ventricle in a symmetrical manner, or it may involve the wall of muscle that separates the left and right ventricles. No matter the location of the thickening, contraction of the ventricle is not usually a problem. In fact, the ventricle may contract exceedingly strongly. Filling of the left ventricle, however, is often abnormal because its elasticity is decreased by the thick muscle. Think of the muscle-bound weightlifter who cannot touch his toes. When the heart is too stiff to fill appropriately, it fails. People with hypertrophic cardiomyopathy may have no symptoms at all. Others have shortness of breath, chest pain, or fainting spells.

Like Amanda's brother, some people will die suddenly, unaware that they even had a heart problem, let alone a potentially deadly one. Whenever I hear of a young athlete who dies suddenly during or shortly after a game, I think of hypertrophic cardiomyopathy. Most people who have this type do well as long as sudden death is prevented. A very few people will develop a dilated cardiomyopathy from a hypertrophic one.

There are multiple genes that may, when abnormal, cause hypertrophic cardiomyopathy. Even within a specific gene, multiple mutations at different sites along the DNA may cause the disease. Not everyone with an abnormal gene will manifest the disease immediately; in fact, most of them will not until at least after puberty. Some will have a normal heart for a long time and then develop the disease much later in life, in their sixties or beyond. A person with a genetic mutation for hypertrophic cardiomyopathy may need to be screened for her entire life.

RESTRICTIVE CARDIOMYOPATHY

Ernesto was 65 years old and had severe heart failure and multiple myeloma—a form of cancer in which the cancer cells make an abnormal and often intrusive protein that is deposited in tissues all over the body. He had a very severe case of amyloidosis—a disorder in which a substance called amyloid protein builds up in the body's organs. Ernesto's amyloidosis included massive deposits of amyloid protein in his heart. Once deposited, the protein cannot be dissolved.

Like many patients with this form of cardiomyopathy, Ernesto died of intractable heart failure within six months of diagnosis. Before he died, he was seldom able to leave his bed. The amyloid protein was also in his liver, kidneys, gut, and skin, so he was not a candidate for heart transplantation because there is no known way to get rid of the amyloid once it is there. These other organs would eventually fail, and the new heart could get amyloid if his body continued to produce it.

In restrictive cardiomyopathy, the ventricles are too stiff to fill with blood as they should. Unlike hypertrophic cardiomyopathy, the walls are not enlarged. The ejection fraction is normal or near normal, and the size of the heart is usually normal. It is the least common of the three main cardiomyopathies. Amyloidosis is the most frequent cause of restrictive cardiomyopathy, but the condition can also be inherited or caused by radiation administered to the chest as a cancer treatment.

People with restrictive cardiomyopathy most often have symptoms of swelling in their legs or abdomen and less commonly have shortness of breath. The heart is simply too stiff to work well as a pump. Restrictive cardiomyopathy is sometimes confused with *constrictive pericarditis,* where the heart is strangled by the sac (*pericardium*) in which it sits. The difference is important, because the abnormal pericardium can be surgically removed in constrictive pericarditis. This procedure will not help people with restrictive cardiomyopathy.

ARRHYTHMOGENIC RIGHT VENTRICULAR DYSPLASIA

Arrhythmogenic right ventricular dysplasia (ARVD) is a rare inherited cardiomyopathy in which the wall of the right ventricle is replaced by fat, and the right ventricle is enlarged. People with this disease usually have rapid heartbeats. Heart failure is rare in people with ARVD, but the condition is included here because it is one of the forms of cardiomyopathy. With ARVD, sudden death, unfortunately, is common—common enough that, to prevent it from rapid wild heartbeats, everyone with this form of cardiomyopathy should get an ICD.

The many variables of cardiomyopathies—causes, symptoms, treatment, and prognosis—are a source of confusion for people with a cardiomyopathy and physicians alike. One thing is certain, however: it is extremely important to ask your doctor what type of cardiomyopathy you have and whether it can run in families. If it is an inheritable type, your family members should get their hearts tested, too.

4

Diagnosing Heart Failure and Its Causes

We all have been through experiences that, in retrospect, were nowhere near as awful as we had anticipated. The CT scan you dreaded or the colonoscopy you endured at age 50—not as bad as you thought they would be, were they? Medical tests are much less intimidating if you know what to expect. In this chapter, we will describe history taking, the physical examination, and commonly performed tests in the diagnosis, evaluation, and management of heart failure.

MEDICAL HISTORY AND PHYSICAL EXAMINATION

First, your doctor will want to explore what has happened to you throughout your life—your complete history. In some instances, supplying specific details and dates will be crucial. Your precise description and clear timeline of illnesses and surgeries will help the doctor make the right diagnosis and create an appropriate treatment plan. For the best outcome, prepare for your visit by writing these details down in advance. That way you will easily and accurately be able to answer questions about your health and medical history. Talk to your family, who can help you remember what you experienced and when. Bring copies of pertinent medical records with you when you see your doctor, or better still, send your records in advance so your doctor can review them before seeing you. When I (Ed) am able to review records in advance, I have more time to spend speaking with my patient.

Your doctor is likely to ask you these questions:

1. *Do you find it hard to breathe normally? When does this shortness of breath, or "air hunger," develop? Only after exercising? Or does it occur after normal activities such as taking a shower or walking from one part of your house to another? When climbing stairs? Even when sitting? When lying down? How many pillows do you sleep on?* There are many causes of shortness of breath and fatigue. Your doctor will want to determine the cause as the very first step. Sometimes, arriving at a diagnosis can be difficult because heart failure can coexist with other disorders that cause shortness of breath, such as emphysema or asthma. In young patients, heart failure may be mistaken for pneumonia or bronchitis.
2. *Do you often feel tired? Do you need to stop and rest your hands on the back of a chair or lean against a wall or sit down as you walk from one part of your house or workplace to another?*
3. *Do you experience chest pain or pressure?*
4. *Do you ever have lightheadedness or fainting spells, a sense that your heart is racing or skipping beats?*
5. *Do you have swelling in your ankles, feet, or abdomen?* Your doctor will also check for swelling during the physical examination.

During the physical exam, the doctor will measure your blood pressure in both arms (especially if you have high blood pressure), take your pulse, and record your weight and height. I spend some time listening to a patient's heart for abnormal heart sounds or murmurs that might indicate a heart problem. I also listen to the lungs for abnormal sounds that indicate fluid in the lungs. I palpate the abdomen to check the liver and find out whether it is swollen with fluid. I pinch the patient's ankles to see if they are retaining fluid. Taking a complete history and doing a thorough physical examination take time. They cannot be done in 15 minutes. Expect this first visit to last as long as an hour.

The diagnosis of heart failure is a *clinical diagnosis,* which means no tests can definitively establish it. Doctors make this diagnosis depending on what the patient tells them and what they find when they examine the patient.

Once the diagnosis of heart failure is made, the next step is to find out, if possible, what caused the heart failure. Again, a complete history and physical examination are critical. In reality, at your first visit your doctor is likely considering a diagnosis of heart failure and beginning to evaluate what caused it. Diagnostic tests can pick up some causes of heart failure: Coronary disease, valvular heart disease, disease of the *pericardium* (the sac containing the heart), and disease of the *myocardium* (the heart muscle itself), which is cardiomyopathy, can only be diagnosed through testing. Other causes of heart failure can be suggested by a thorough medical history and generally can be confirmed through medical testing. These causes include diabetes, thyroid disease and other hormonal problems, overuse of alcohol, use of cocaine and other street drugs, some prescription drugs (see the sidebars in this chapter), lupus, HIV, and hereditary or genetic causes. By the time I have finished taking the patient's history during the very first visit, I have created in my head a list of possible causes of the heart failure. In the search for a cause, I ask six sets of questions at that first visit.

1. *Have you had or do you now have high blood pressure, diabetes mellitus, high cholesterol?*
2. *Do you smoke? If so, for how long and how frequently?* If you smoke, you should stop.
3. *Do you drink alcohol? If so, how much and how often? Do you use any kind of nonprescription drugs?* Certain over-the-counter herbal remedies can be toxic to the heart, such as those containing ephedra. You may find it intrusive to be asked about alcohol and drug use, but honesty helps your doctor both make the correct diagnosis and begin proper therapy.
4. *Have you ever had heart disease, even as a child?*
5. *Have you ever had cancer? If so, how was this treated?* Some of the drugs used to treat cancer may cause dilated cardiomyopathy, which leads to heart failure. Radiation therapy to the chest can also injure the heart.
6. *Have you had thyroid problems, obesity, or nutritional disorders?* Your doctor will want to discuss with you how these disorders were treated and whether the therapy was successful.

Bring a list of your medications, including the dose and how many times a day you take your medicines. Some patients find it easier to just put all their medication bottles into a bag and bring it to the doctor's office. Whether you bring the medicines themselves or a list of them, remember to include any over-the-counter drugs, herbal remedies, and nutritional supplements. Also bring a list of medications or supplements you have taken in the past, including those not prescribed by your doctor.

You will be asked about your family because both coronary disease and cardiomyopathy can run in families. Attention to detail is critical.

Drugs That Commonly Cause Heart Failure or Make It Worse
Drugs to Avoid or to Use with Caution

Many drugs may cause or worsen heart failure, yet they are absolutely essential in the treatment of diseases like cancer and depression. In the following list, drugs that are starred (*) should be avoided by people with heart failure, but most of these drugs are not to be avoided as much as used carefully, while being alert for the development of heart failure symptoms. As always, make your doctor aware of all medications and supplements you are using, whether by prescription or over the counter.

- **Alcohol—only when used in excess. Exception: If your cardiomyopathy was caused by alcohol use, avoid drinking alcohol.**
- **Amphetamines and catecholamines**
- **Anticancer drugs—anthracyclines, capecitabine, cyclophosphamide, 5-fluorouracil, mitoxantrone, trastuzumab**
- **Antidepressants—most tricyclic antidepressants**
- **Antifungal drugs—itraconazole, amphotericine B**
- **Antimigrane drugs—ergotamine, methysergide**
- **Antipsychotic drugs—clozapine**
- ***Cocaine—recreational use should be avoided. It is sometimes used as an anesthetic agent in nose surgery.**
- ***Ephedra, other Chinese herbal supplements containing licorice—not good for anyone.**
- **Immune system modifiers—etanercept, imatinib, infliximab, interferon-alpha-2, interleukin-2**
- **Lithium**
- **Almost any drug can cause an allergic reaction, which in turn may cause cardiomyopathy. Most common are antibiotics.**

Drugs That Cause Fluid Retention and Worsen Heart Failure

Certain drugs may worsen the fluid retention that is so much a part of heart failure. Most of these drugs have alternatives. Discuss with your doctor the possible use of alternative drugs if you have heart failure and you take any of these medications.

- **Calcium channel blockers—nifedipine, diltazem, verapamil. Avoid these drugs if you have heart failure due to a weakened heart muscle. These drugs may be used in people with heart failure and normal heart function.**
- **Nonsteroidal anti-inflammatory drugs (NSAIDs), including cyclooxygenase-2 inhibitors (COX-2 inhibitors). Avoid all, including ibuprofen. May be used but very carefully in patients with heart failure. Close monitoring of kidney function is essential.**
- **Antidiabetic drugs—pioglitazone, rosiglitazone. Should probably be avoided in people with heart failure.**
- **Glucocorticoids. Avoid all. May need to be used despite heart failure if no good alternative exists.**

Your family may believe that your father died of a heart attack, for example, but he may have died suddenly with a dilated cardiomyopathy instead. These are two very different things. The term "heart attack" has a very specific meaning to your doctor, and not everyone who dies suddenly died of a heart attack. The term "heart problems" is not specific enough to help your doctor understand your risk of an inherited disorder, so you need to gather as much information as you can about heart disease in your family. For instance, you may be able to get death certificates of your grandparents. Write down what you find out and bring the written information to your doctor.

DIAGNOSTIC TESTS

Diagnostic tests are done to learn the cause of heart failure and are useful in ruling out other causes of the patient's symptoms.

Blood Tests

Expect some blood to be drawn from a vein in your arm. Several tubes of blood will be taken to measure kidney and liver function, your white and red blood cell counts, and your cholesterol. Urine should be obtained to evaluate kidney function. If your doctor has a reason to do so based on findings from your medical history and physical examination, several other blood tests may be ordered, such as a test to measure thyroid function or to detect the presence of HIV antibody.

A BNP or a proBNP test is likely. BNP is short for *brain natriuretic peptide*, a protein the heart produces when under a major stress such as a heart attack or heart failure. ProBNP is the precursor. An elevated BNP or proBNP is associated with progressive heart failure. Age, gender, weight, and kidney function may influence BNP levels. This test is often used in the emergency room if there is a question of whether a heart problem or a lung problem is causing shortness of breath.

Chest X-ray

An x-ray of the chest is a way to confirm a diagnosis of heart failure, but the x-ray may be relatively normal even in the presence of the condition. Alternatively, the chest x-ray may show significant disease, even if you are responding nicely to treatment. Chest x-rays tend to lag behind improvement in symptoms. They are done both to confirm the presence of heart failure and to make sure that other lung problems, such as pneumonia, are not present. In heart failure, the lungs, which appear black in a normal x-ray, have a hazy white appearance because fluid is occupying the lung spaces.

Echocardiogram

Using sound waves to take images of how the heart is working in real time, an *echocardiogram* ("echo" for short), is the single most useful test in looking for the cause of heart failure (figure 4.1). (This is the same technology that is used to visualize the fetus in a pregnant woman.) As you lie on a table with a pillow under your head, a technician places electrodes on your chest and ribs and presses a scanning device against your left chest, moving it to different parts of the heart. The echo looks at the structure and function of your heart to detect abnormalities that cause

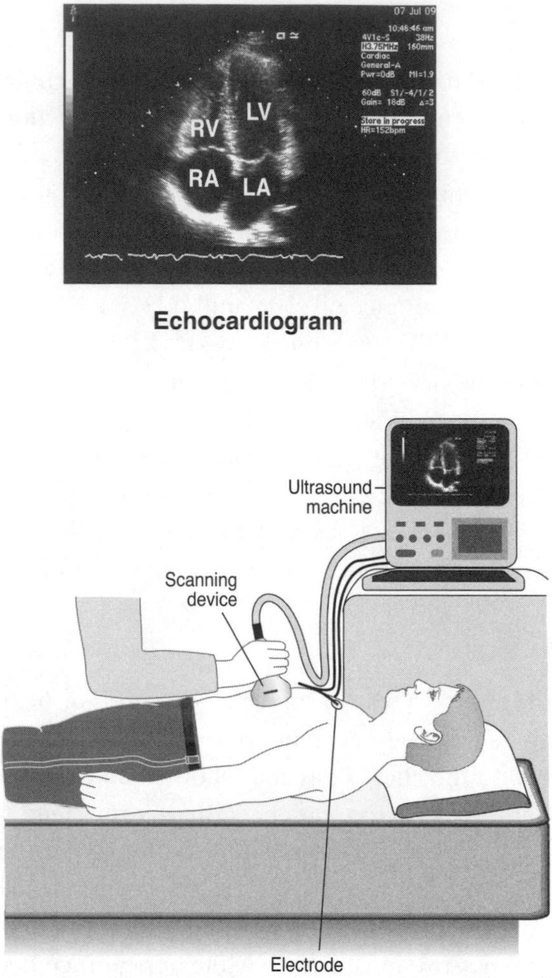

Figure 4.1. Echocardiography. A variety of different pictures can be generated depending on the location of the scanning device on the chest. This is probably the single most useful test in the evaluation of heart failure.

the signs and symptoms that we call heart failure. You can watch your heart beating on a TV screen as the technician is performing the test.

An echo shows how strongly your heart beats by giving its ejection fraction, or EF, an estimate of how well your left ventricle is contracting. A normal EF is considered greater than 55 percent, which means that the left ventricle is pushing out 55 percent of the blood in its chamber with each heartbeat. An echo also provides information about the size of your heart (for instance, whether the left ventricle has become enlarged), how well your heart valves open and shut, and some information about the pericardium. Echocardiography is the key to understanding whether there is damage to your heart and, if so, how severe it is. This test is painless, or nearly so. Women may find that the pressure of the scanning instrument against the chest causes discomfort similar to that of a mammogram. But the test does not include exposure to radiation, does not require you to slide into a tube (as for an MRI), and can be done quickly. Echocardiography is the single most important test to perform after a good history and physical examination.

Electrocardiogram

This two-minute painless test records the electrical activity of your heart through electrodes placed on your chest, arms, and legs while you are lying down. An *electrocardiogram* (ECG or EKG; figure 4.2) can find evidence of prior myocardial infarctions or abnormal heart rhythms.

TESTS FOR CORONARY ARTERY DISEASE

If you are diagnosed with heart failure, your doctor will want to find out whether you have coronary artery disease, which (as discussed in chapter 2) can cause heart failure. Coronary artery disease can be treated. To determine whether you have this disease and which arteries are blocked with fatty deposits, you may have a stress test, a cardiac catheterization, or the newer test, called coronary CT angiogram.

Stress Testing

Stress testing is a way to see how your heart functions under stressful conditions (figure 4.3). Asking the patient to walk on a treadmill is the usual manner of administering this test. Tell your doctor if you think that you will not be able to walk on a treadmill, because you don't feel steady on your feet, because you are afraid of the treadmill, or for any other reason.

You will be asked not to eat or drink anything for at least four hours prior to the test. Since you will be asked to walk on a treadmill, you need to arrive at the testing site prepared to walk, with comfortable shoes and

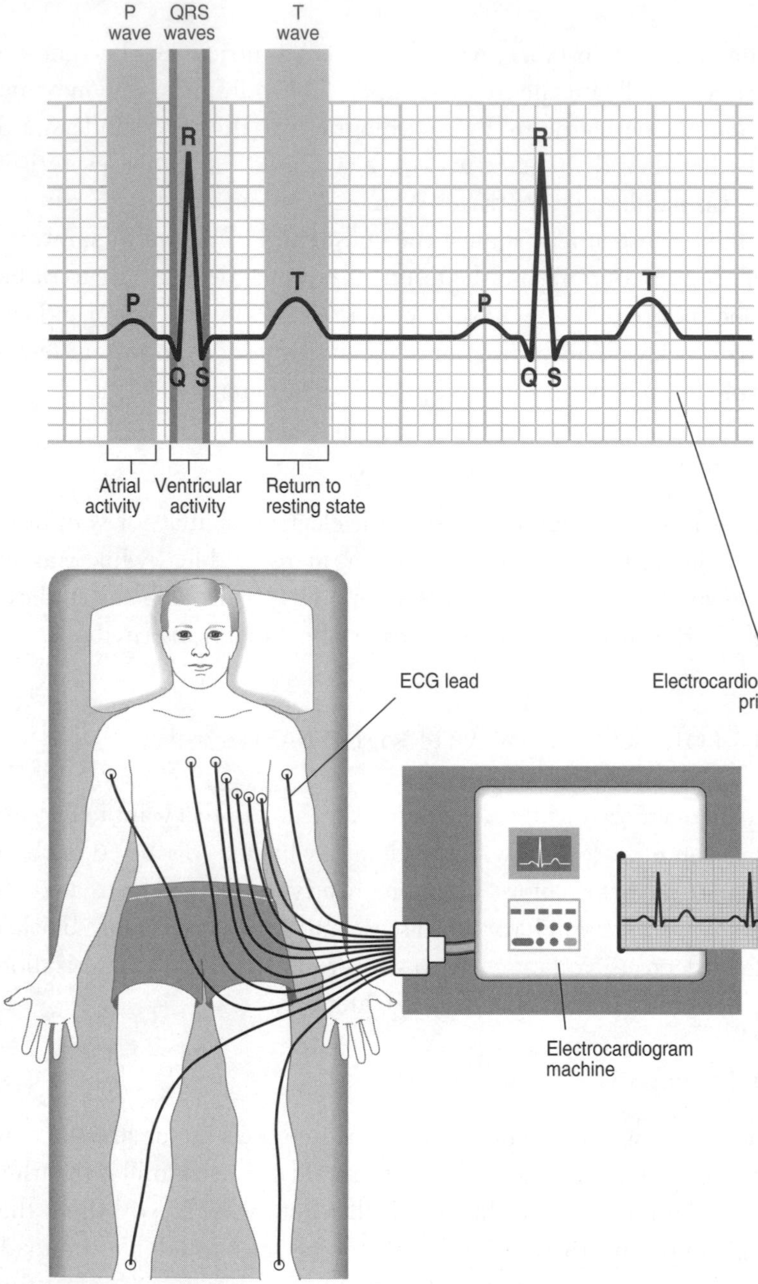

Figure 4.2. Electrocardiography (ECG). The electrocardiogram machine measures the electrical activity of the heart. The P wave results from atrial activation. The QRS represents ventricular electrical activity. The T wave represents a return to the baseline electrical state of the ventricles. Without electrical activity in a coordinated fashion, the heart will not function correctly.

clothing that allows easy movement. The treadmill will start slowly and then gradually increase in both speed and incline. You will be connected to an ECG, and your blood pressure will be taken frequently before, during, and after exercising. You should exercise for as long as you can or until the person supervising your test tells you to stop.

Expect to get a good workout; you will be sweating and short of breath by the time you are finished. If you develop shortness of breath, chest pain, pressure, or lightheadedness, immediately tell the person supervising the test. If you feel unsafe for any reason, feel free to speak up and say you want to stop. Although exercise is the preferred "stress,"

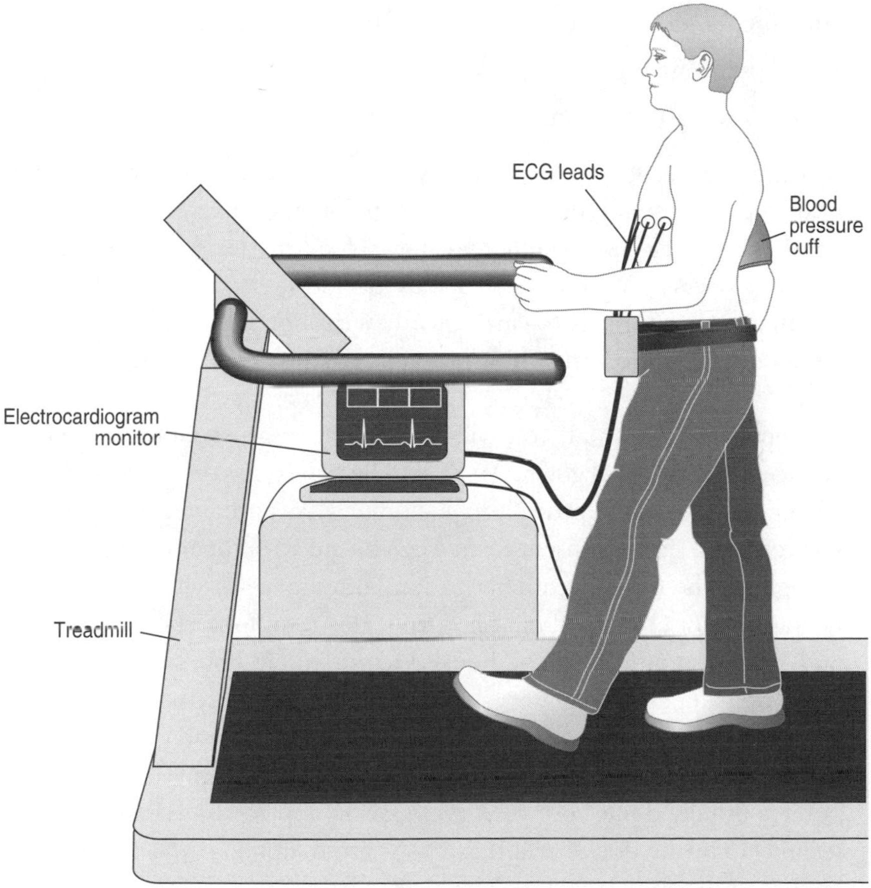

Figure 4.3. Exercise stress testing. This test is typically done on a treadmill. For those who cannot walk, drugs may be used to simulate the results of exercise.

various drugs can be used to mimic exercise. Your doctor may want to add echocardiography or a nuclear scan as you do the stress test, to get more detailed information. A *nuclear scan* uses a small amount of radioactive material to examine both blood flow to the heart and how well your heart is contracting.

Exercise stress testing can also be combined with measurement of oxygen consumption and carbon dioxide production. To do this testing, you are asked to breathe through a mouthpiece similar to the kind of mouthpiece that is used for snorkeling. Measurement of oxygen consumption during exercise offers a good measure of prognosis in patients with heart failure due to dilated cardiomyopathy. The medical term for this test is *metabolic stress testing*, or *cardiopulmonary stress testing*. This test is often used to decide which patients are so sick that they should be considered for a heart transplant.

Cardiac Catheterization, or Angiogram

If a stress test suggests that you may have coronary artery disease, the next step will usually be *cardiac catheterization* (also called an *angiogram*), which will show clearly whether you have blocked arteries and the extent of any blockage. Your physician may decide to skip stress testing altogether and go directly to cardiac catheterization. You will be asked to fast (not to eat or drink anything) for at least eight hours before a cardiac "cath."

Once at the hospital, you will be brought to a preparation area to change into a hospital gown. An IV will be placed in your arm, and you will be told about the procedure, including risks and alternatives. After you read and sign a consent form to go ahead with the test, you will be brought to the cardiac catheterization laboratory, which resembles an operating room. You will be asked to lie down on a hard narrow table, and various monitors will be hooked to you, including an ECG and a blood pressure cuff. Bright overhead lights shine on you to help the doctor see during the test.

A cardiac catheterization can be done from either an arm or a leg, but it is usually done from your groin, at the top of your right thigh. A technician or the doctor will shave your groin area and wash it with an antibacterial solution. You will be given a light sedative—not enough to put you to sleep, but enough to relax you. If you feel chilly, technicians or nurses can cover you with a warmed blanket.

Using a needle, the doctor will then numb the skin over the right femoral artery (or the brachial artery in the arm) by injecting an anesthetic drug such as lidocaine. Using a different needle, the doctor will place a plastic sheath that will serve as a tunnel into the right femoral artery, which has a circumference the size of your index finger. The sheath is an entry device for a catheter, tubing not much larger than a piece of spaghetti, which your doctor will push up to your coronary arteries and into the mouth of each coronary artery, one at a time. Dye is injected through the catheter down your coronary arteries to reveal any blockages. This test involves exposure to radiation and takes about 30 minutes. (See figure 4.4.)

After the catheterization is complete, the catheter and the sheath will be removed. Pressure will be applied to your groin to prevent bleeding. You will then go to a recovery room, where you will lie flat for 2 to 3 hours, then sit up for a while and finally get up and walk around. You will be observed to make sure that everything is fine and that there is no bleeding. Unless a problem occurred, you will go home the same day. Someone must drive you home after the procedure. For at least 48 hours after you get home, do not squat or pick up anything heavy. You can drive within 24 hours of the procedure.

There are risks to cardiac catheterization, which you should discuss with your doctor. The most feared complications are stroke, heart attack, and death. There is about a 1 in 1,000 chance that one of these events will occur. They are a risk because the catheter is pushed through the artery, which can damage the artery, and because the catheter is pushed up to the heart, which can damage the aorta. Usually, the patient's degree of risk for one of these events relates to how sick the patient is before the cardiac catheterization.

Some people are allergic to the dye used to outline the inside of the coronary arteries. Most people with a dye allergy can undergo cardiac catheterization, but they *must* be treated first with drugs intended to prevent the allergic response. It is most important to let your doctor know in advance of taking this test if you have a dye allergy. However, I (Mary) caution that I have a dye allergy and told the doctor in advance of getting an angiogram and took the drugs intended to prevent an allergic response. Yet I died on the table and had to be resuscitated with four electric shocks. Always weigh the benefit and the potential harm before agreeing to take any medical test.

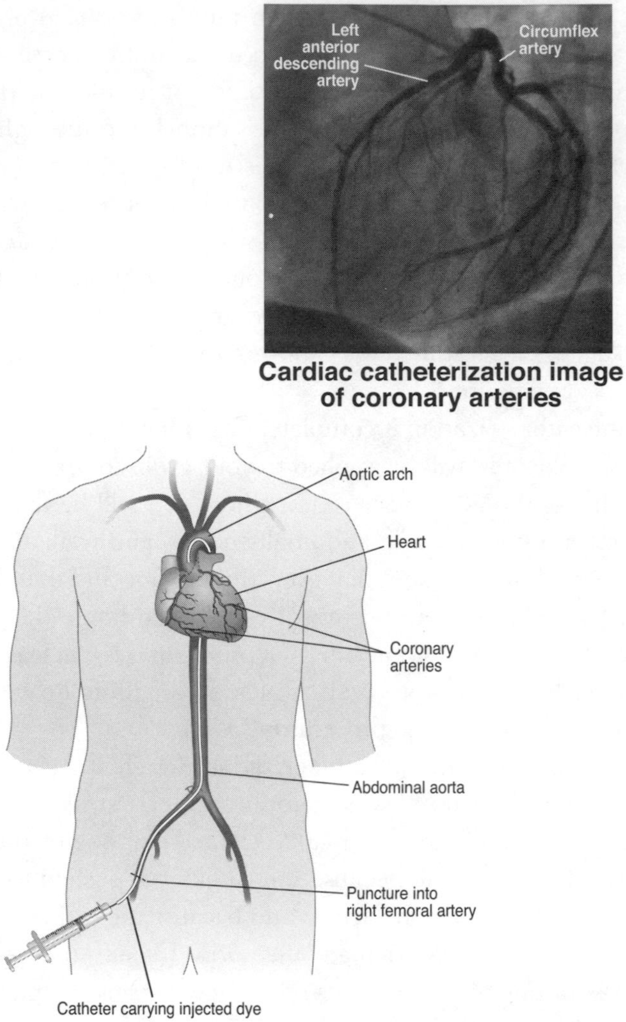

Figure 4.4. Cardiac catheterization, or coronary arteriography. Images of the insides of coronary arteries are generated during cardiac catheterization. This allows the number and degree of coronary blockages to be determined. Armed with this road map, doctors can decide how best to treat the patient.

Rarely, the dye can cause kidney problems, especially if you already have kidney problems to begin with. Doctors can minimize this risk by giving the least amount of dye possible and by giving some medications and IV fluids immediately before the cardiac catheterization that flush the kidneys to prevent buildup of the dye in them. This pretreatment of the kidneys is not routinely done, and you may want to ask your doctor if you can receive it to help prevent kidney damage.

Cardiac catheterization provides a road map of the coronary arteries. Using the road map, your doctor can make a decision about what needs to be done next, if anything, and how it can best be done. Medications and lifestyle changes may be enough treatment. Other treatments include stenting to push aside the blockage, or coronary artery bypass grafting (CABG), commonly known as bypass surgery. Stenting is less often a treatment of choice for stable coronary artery disease because of the findings of a huge clinical study reported in 2007. But when stenting is necessary, it often is done at the same time as cardiac catheterization. We discuss treatment options for coronary artery disease and angina in chapter 2.

Coronary CT Angiogram

A newer alternative to cardiac catheterization is a special type of CT scan called a *coronary CT angiogram*. The scan produces detailed 3-D pictures of the coronary arteries. This type of study is also done with dye injected through an IV placed in your arm, and it also includes exposure to radiation (see figure 4.5). A 2007 study at fifty university and community hospitals found that radiation doses varied significantly, with the median dose the equivalent of 600 chest x-rays. You will lie down on a narrow table that will be rolled into a tube so that the upper half of your body is inside the machine. The good part about this test is that all the needed pictures can be taken during a single 10-second period. You will be asked to hold your breath for these 10 seconds to still the motion of your breathing, which would disturb the images.

In addition to pictures of the coronary arteries, a coronary CT angiogram provides detailed information about the structure and function of your heart, much like an echocardiogram. The advantage of CT angiography is avoiding a stick in the femoral artery and a catheter being pushed up to the coronary arteries. Recovery from CT angiography is immediate, and you do not have to stay for observation after this study. You can drive yourself home or back to work. The risk of a harmful event occurring during this test is less than 1 in 10,000. The risk is lower than in an angiogram (cardiac catheterization) because no artery is entered, so no artery can be ruptured. No catheter is pushed up to the

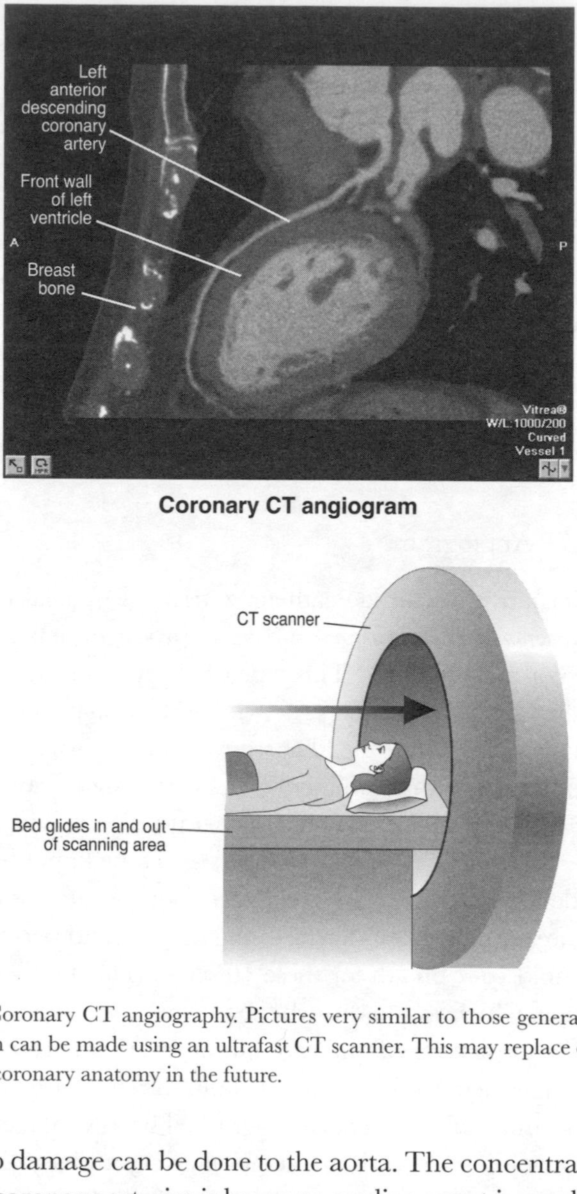

Figure 4.5. Coronary CT angiography. Pictures very similar to those generated at cardiac catheterization can be made using an ultrafast CT scanner. This may replace cardiac catheterization for coronary anatomy in the future.

heart, so no damage can be done to the aorta. The concentration of dye within the coronary arteries is lower, so cardiac arrest is much less likely. However, the radiation dose is higher. Ed points out that the newest models of CT angiogram scanners have reduced the dose of radiation, and he thinks CT angiography will replace most cardiac catheterization in the near future. Mary remains cautious about both tests and points out that the many hospitals and doctor groups who already bought earlier models of these very expensive machines will not throw them away and rush out to buy the newest model.

We both advise you to ask questions, including how much radiation you would get from the CT angiogram scanner that would be used for your test, before agreeing to have one.

Heart Biopsy

Rarely, it is necessary to biopsy the heart, a procedure that is easier than it sounds. A biopsy is performed when your doctor thinks that something, such as an abnormal protein or inflammatory cells, is infiltrating your heart. The biopsy is most often done in a setting much like that described for a cardiac catheterization. The procedure is usually done from the right internal jugular vein in the right side of your neck. Using local numbing medication, your doctor inserts a sheath into the right internal jugular vein. Through the sheath, a surgical instrument called a *bioptome,* which looks rather like a long pair of tweezers, is pushed along the vein and into the right ventricle of the heart under x-ray guidance. Echocardiography may be used to guide placement of the bioptome in the right ventricle. Several small pieces of the heart are clipped off to examine under the microscope to look for the cause of your cardiomyopathy.

Normally the physician samples only the right ventricle because it is safer. To sample the right ventricle, there is no need to enter an artery; the procedure involves only the veins and the right side of the heart, where the pressure is lower. The right ventricle reflects what is going on in the left ventricle. This procedure takes about 30 minutes. Then you spend about an hour or less in a recovery room and can go home or back to work. You can drive yourself.

If you have been diagnosed with heart failure, discuss your options with your doctor, including any alternative tests as well as risks associated with each test. Get all your questions answered. A doctor who will not spend the time to answer your questions is unlikely to be the right doctor for you. Although there are situations when things must be done emergently, when time is of the essence, most often there is time for questions and answers. You should feel comfortable with your decision before going forward, because it is your body and your health. The more you know, the easier it will be to make the right decision and to undergo the procedure because you will know what to expect.

Part II

TREATMENTS *for* HEART FAILURE

5

Drug Treatments

Drug therapy is the cornerstone of heart failure management. Many people with heart failure who take not only the right drugs, but also the right doses of the right drugs, can enjoy a longer life with decreased symptoms and fewer or no hospitalizations for heart failure. In fact, some people can recover completely from the condition. So, it is crucial to be on the right drug treatments. If you are not taking the medications discussed in this chapter, ask your doctor if there is a reason you cannot take them. If there is no reason, you may want to ask about switching to these drugs.

The rationale behind drug therapy for heart failure is scientific knowledge about the cycle that takes place in a person's body once the heart begins to fail. When the heart starts falling behind in pumping blood to the body, nerves that react to stress respond with an outpouring of *neurohormones*. These chemicals are intended to boost the heart's performance so the body can get the full amount of blood it needs, but, as described in chapter 1, these chemicals can damage the heart instead. You need help eliminating the excess stimulation. Medications do this by blocking the hormonal stimulation and easing the heart's workload.

This cycle—weakened heart, response of outpouring hormones, continued weakened heart, more hormonal drenching—is the basis for current guidelines on first-line medicines for heart failure. The American College of Cardiology (ACC) and the American Heart Association (AHA) appointed a joint committee to review reports of drug treatment clinical trials in the medical literature and to recommend guidelines for treating heart failure. *The American College of Cardiology /American Heart Association Guidelines for the Evaluation and Management of Chronic Heart Failure in the Adult* (ACC /AHA Guidelines) are the gold standard of care for treating heart failure. The full text of these recommendations can be found on the ACC and AHA Web sites: www.acc.org and www.americanheart.org. The tables that appear in this chapter are based on these guidelines.

The ACC and AHA are not the only organizations with published recommendations for the diagnosis and treatment of people with heart failure. The Heart Failure Society of America (HFSA) and the European Society of Cardiology (ESC) have issued excellent guidelines as well. There is remarkable agreement on major recommendations among all of them.

In this chapter I (Ed) describe my approach to the management of heart failure as informed by all three major guidelines—ACC /AHA, HFSA, and ESC—as well as my own reading of the medical literature and my experience caring for people with heart failure over the last 15 years.

If the most respected organizations of heart specialists meet and review the drug studies in medical journals, discuss the findings, and issue guidelines on what drugs to prescribe for different types of heart failure, you may think that all doctors will follow the recommendations and that all patients will take the most effective drugs. But studies have shown that this does not always happen. For various reasons, many doctors do not always follow the guidelines. That is why you need to find out if you are taking the drugs listed in this chapter for your type of heart failure. If not, ask your doctor why not. There may or may not be a valid reason, and you will only find out by asking. You want to be sure you are getting the benefit of all currently recommended treatments for heart failure that are safe for you to take, given your medical history and current condition. These guidelines are a tool to manage the condition of people at risk for heart failure and people with heart failure. The recommendations are updated regularly, every 4 or 5 years and as major research trials are published that change the way doctors care for people with heart failure. Guidelines are based not only on research but also on the opinions of physicians who are expert in the management of patients with heart failure. In general, physicians learn about new guidelines by reading the medical literature and attending scientific conferences.

The guidelines recommend two major categories of drugs—*ACE inhibitors* and *beta blockers*—for most types of heart failure, because many clinical trials and animal experiments have shown that these medications block or otherwise prevent much of the action of the hormones that harm the heart.

ACE inhibitors do just what their name says. They inhibit the action of *angiotensin-converting enzyme* (ACE). Stopping this enzyme from acting is important because it otherwise changes a precursor hormone called *angiotensin I* into the active hormone *angiotensin II*, the one that damages the heart.

Beta blockers work differently but are equally important. On the heart muscle and on many other cells are receptors for *norepinephrine*, the adrenalinelike hormone. When the hormone binds to those receptors, it turns on cascades of enzymes within the cell, much like when you pass your hand in front of an automatic faucet and the water comes on. Beta-blocker drugs cover the receptors like a plug of putty, preventing the hormones from entering. ACE inhibitors and beta blockers not only stop the onslaught of hormones; they can actually remodel a heart that grew too large and out of shape as it struggled to send an adequate blood supply to the body.

These drugs were found to work in clinical trials in which a large number of patients randomly received either the drug being tested or a placebo pill containing no drug, only an inert ingredient. To judge how effective a new drug is, it must be compared either to the old drug it will replace or to a placebo. The best of these clinical trials were also *double blinded*, meaning that neither the patients nor their doctors knew whether the patients were taking the active drug or the placebo. Blind testing is done to minimize bias—the preconceived idea of both patients and doctors that the new drug being tested might be either better or worse than the older drug or than the placebo to which it is being compared. Randomized, double-blind, placebo-controlled clinical trials are responsible for the remarkable improvement in survival of patients with many medical problems, including heart failure. (The principal clinical trials that are the basis for these recommendations are summarized in the Notes on Sources.)

Some clinical trials refer to patients' *ejection fraction*, which is a method of categorizing the severity of the heart muscle's weakness. A normal ejection fraction is between 55 percent and 65 percent. This means that about 60 percent of the blood in the left ventricle is pumped out with the beginning of each contraction or heartbeat. An ejection fraction of less than 50 percent is abnormal.

In this chapter, we refer to drugs by their generic (or scientific) name rather than by the trade (or brand) name that the pharmaceutical company uses. A generic name helps avoid confusion because the drug has the same generic name regardless of which drug company produces it. (Each of the drug companies gives the drug a different brand name, and it is one of these brand names that you will typically see on your medication bottle.) Use of generic names also avoids promoting any particular drug company's brand. A list of commonly used drugs giving both their generic and brand names can be found in the appendix.

As discussed in chapter 3, there are many causes of heart failure, some that make a heart weak and some that do not. The medical term for a weakened heart muscle is *left ventricular systolic dysfunction*, or simply *systolic dysfunction*. "Systolic" refers to the contraction of the heart when it pumps blood out to the body, and "dysfunction" means the contraction is not as strong as it should be. A person with an ejection fraction under 50 percent has systolic dysfunction, a weakened heart. The term *nonsystolic heart failure* refers to a condition in which the heart is not weak—the person has a normal ejection fraction greater than 55 percent. Heart failure caused by a weak heart is treated differently from heart failure that occurs with a normally contracting heart.

These are the three categories of heart failure:

1. Weakened heart with no symptoms of heart failure
2. Weakened heart with symptoms of heart failure
3. Heart failure with a normally contracting heart

In the rest of this chapter, we discuss drugs used for each kind of heart failure, followed by sections describing the proper doses, risks, and side effects of these drugs. Many drugs are discussed here—so many that you may want to skim the chapter to find your type of heart failure and read the recommendations for your type.

WEAKENED HEART WITH NO SYMPTOMS OF HEART FAILURE

Perhaps half of all people who have developed a weakened heart muscle, or systolic dysfunction, have no symptoms. If you have been diagnosed with systolic dysfunction but have no symptoms of heart failure, the condition was probably discovered serendipitously when an echocardiogram was done to evaluate another problem. To say your diagnosis is a surprise is an understatement! But you can also feel lucky or thankful that the problem was caught early, because although you feel well and are not experiencing the characteristic symptoms of heart failure, you are at significant risk for developing it.

As soon as you are diagnosed your doctor should get you started on a combination of an ACE inhibitor and a beta blocker and stop the treatment or lower the dose of the drugs only if you experience significant side effects. You should be taking the same doses of ACE inhibitor and beta blocker that are listed below, under "Weakened Heart with Symptoms of Heart Failure." The same risks and side effects apply as well.

WEAKENED HEART WITH SYMPTOMS OF HEART FAILURE

When a person has heart failure with symptoms (see chapter 1), the following medications are recommended: ACE inhibitor, beta blocker, loop diuretic, possibly digoxin, and spironolactone for moderate or severe heart failure. Those who cannot tolerate an ACE inhibitor may be prescribed an angiotensin receptor blocker instead.

ACE Inhibitors

If you have a weakened heart with symptoms, you should try to reach the higher doses of ACE inhibitors used in clinical trials. If you can't tolerate the high doses, however, ACC/AHA guidelines advise doctors to prescribe low doses of an ACE inhibitor "with the expectation that there are likely to be only small differences in efficacy between low and high doses." You begin on a low dose of an ACE inhibitor to prevent side effects, and the dose is increased every one to two weeks until the target dose is reached or until side effects occur (table 5.1). I find that most people tolerate ACE inhibitors well.

Angiotensin Receptor Blockers

People who cannot tolerate an ACE inhibitor, usually because it causes a frequent dry cough, are prescribed an *angiotensin receptor blocker* (ARB) instead. Angiotensin II works by binding to receptors on many different

Table 5.1. ACE Inhibitors (Generic)

ACE inhibitor	*Starting dose*	*Target dose*
Captopril	6.25 mg 3 times a day	50 mg 3 times a day
Enalapril	2.5 mg twice daily	10 mg twice daily
Fosinopril	5 mg once daily	40 mg once daily
Lisinopril	2.5 mg once daily	20 to 40 mg once daily
Quinapril	10 mg twice daily	40 mg twice daily
Ramipril	1.25 mg once daily	10 mg once daily

types of cells. Angiotensin receptor blockers bind to the receptors and block angiotensin II from interacting with its receptor.

Remember that ACE inhibitors work by preventing the angiotensin-converting enzyme from changing inactive angiotensin I into active angiotensin II. But now there is evidence that angiotensin II can be created from angiotensin I by enzymes other than the angiotensin-converting enzyme. Not only do ARBs block angiotensin II from its receptor, in clinical trials ARBs appear to be as effective as ACE inhibitors.

People who don't tolerate ACE inhibitors should take an ARB. In addition, if you are already taking an ACE inhibitor and a beta blocker, ask your doctor about adding an ARB if your blood pressure will allow its addition.

Beta Blockers

As of 2009, two beta blockers are approved for use in heart failure by the federal Food and Drug Administration (FDA). They are carvedilol and metoprolol succinate, the long-acting form of metoprolol. These two drugs have never been compared head to head in a clinical trial. Given that there has been no fair test between the two, either one is used in people with heart failure. Bisoprolol, another beta blocker, is widely used in Europe for heart failure, but it has not been approved by the FDA for this purpose.

The dose of the beta blocker matters. Clinical trials have provided good evidence that people in this category of heart failure should be on the highest dose of beta blocker they can tolerate. Generally, a beta blocker is started at a low dose, and this dose is slowly increased to the target dose over several months or until side effects occur (table 5.2). You will ordinarily take an ACE inhibitor before starting the beta blocker,

Table 5.2. Beta Blockers (Generic)

Drug	*Starting dose*	*Target dose*
Carvedilol	3.125 mg twice daily	25–50 mg twice daily
Metoprolol succinate	12.5 mg once daily	200 mg once daily
Bisoprolol*	1.25 mg once daily	10 mg once daily

*Although bisoprolol is not approved by the FDA for treating heart failure, good data exist to support its use in heart failure.

because that is what was done in the clinical trials. I find that most people also tolerate beta blockers well. If one of my patients cannot tolerate the recommended doses of both an ACE inhibitor and a beta blocker, I would rather have the person take a modest dose of both rather than a high dose of the ACE inhibitor and a small dose of the beta blocker. Moderate doses of both seem to work better.

Loop Diuretics

In heart failure, the body retains fluid, causing swelling known as edema, usually located in areas that are low. When a person is standing, this would be the feet and ankles. If a person spends most of the day in bed, this would be the back. Fluid also collects in the lungs, causing shortness of breath, and in the abdomen, leading to bloating and poor appetite.

The kidney acts as a filter, directing sodium and water from the bloodstream into the urine. The kidney then reabsorbs from the urine some of the sodium and water it placed there. How much the kidney reabsorbs depends on how much water and sodium the body needs. If a person sweats during exercise, the body reabsorbs more sodium and water and makes concentrated, yellow urine. If a person has just drunk a lot of water, the kidney reabsorbs less sodium and water and makes dilute, clear urine. Caffeine is a mild natural diuretic, and after drinking a caffeinated beverage such as coffee or cola, a person makes clear, dilute urine.

Fluid retention in heart failure is another example of the body's misguided attempt to compensate for what's wrong. Initially, fluid retention maintains blood pressure. However, over time, fluid retention becomes detrimental, producing many of the symptoms of heart failure and causing high blood pressure. Diuretics are used to produce urine, eliminating this excess fluid and controlling symptoms.

The term *loop diuretic* means the diuretic works in the kidney on the loop of Henle, the part of the kidney where much of the sodium and water is reabsorbed. There is no good alternative to loop diuretics in the management of fluid retention. As people with heart failure know, shortness of breath and edema limit your ability to do the things you want to do, and getting relief from these symptoms is important.

Most people with heart failure will take a loop diuretic such as furosemide, bumetanide, or torsemide. The dose of the diuretic depends largely on the symptoms; it is increased until the person urinates. Even after the excess fluid has been cleared from the body, a diuretic will be continued, at least for a time, to prevent the reaccumulation of fluid. The dose may be modified—increased if too much fluid again accumulates, or decreased if the person taking it becomes dehydrated.

While taking a diuretic, be sure to have your blood tested periodically for potassium and magnesium levels. Loop diuretics cause loss of these electrolytes along with the extra sodium and fluid. Therefore, it is essential to check their levels periodically, and supplement them if necessary. However, do not take potassium or magnesium supplements or try to eat foods high in these elements without first getting this action approved by your doctor. You may be taking another medication that counteracts the potassium loss caused by the first drug. It's just as harmful to get too much as too little potassium in your body.

In heart failure due to systolic dysfunction, diuretics are not used alone. They are used in combination with ACE inhibitors and beta blockers. The ACE inhibitors and beta blockers improve survival and decrease symptoms, while the diuretics only decrease symptoms. That's why people with systolic dysfunction who have no symptoms of heart failure don't need diuretics.

Digoxin

Digoxin or a similar preparation from the foxglove plant has been used for over 200 years. Digoxin decreases the need for hospitalization when heart failure is due to systolic dysfunction. However, a large trial of 6,800 patients found in 1997 that there was no difference in mortality between those in the study who took digoxin and those who took a placebo. Because of this, digoxin, like diuretics, is used only by people who have symptoms of heart failure such as shortness of breath. If the patient's symptoms can be controlled with an ACE inhibitor, beta blocker, and loop diuretic, I do not prescribe digoxin.

The dose of digoxin is usually between 0.125 mg and 0.25 mg once a day. In older and smaller people, a lower dose may be used. Large doses of digoxin are not as effective as smaller doses in the treatment of heart failure and may even worsen heart failure and increase mortality. This is only one extreme example of the importance of not only being on the right drug but also being on the right dose and taking the drug only when it is really needed.

HEART FAILURE WITH A NORMALLY CONTRACTING HEART

Only a few clinical trials have been done to guide the therapy of people who have heart failure despite having a normal or even above normal ejection fraction, proof that their heart is contracting normally and is not weakened. This is nonsystolic heart failure, which most often affects elderly women.

Years of high blood pressure appear to lead to heart failure with normal ejection fraction by causing a stiff heart that does not relax well between beats and so does not fill appropriately with blood. This low reservoir of blood, not a weak heart muscle, prevents an adequate blood supply from moving out to the rest of the body. High blood pressure causes a stiff heart in much the same way that weightlifting may cause stronger but less flexible muscles. The "weight" in this case is the blood pressure against which the heart has to work. So drugs that lower blood pressure, such as candesartan, an angiotensin receptor blocker, are an excellent choice of treatment.

When the heart is stiff, a second goal in therapy is to slow the heartbeat so the heart has more time to fill between beats. Based on clinical experience, but no studies, I have found that drugs such as beta blockers and calcium blockers, which lower the heart rate and cause a slow heartbeat, can also be effective.

The third part of therapy is often a loop diuretic such as furosemide to relieve fluid retention. Beyond these suggestions, there is very little evidence that one drug works better than another. Often, a combination of drugs must be tailored to the individual patient. (These drugs are discussed above, in the section on "Weakened Heart with Symptoms of Heart Failure," and below, under "Drugs to Avoid or Use with Great Care in Certain Populations.")

RISKS AND SIDE EFFECTS OF DRUGS

All drugs have risks and side effects that must be weighed against the proven benefit of each medicine you take. It is very important to have all your prescriptions filled at one pharmacy so the pharmacist can monitor all the drugs you take and check for drug interactions. Every pharmacy is legally required to use a drug interaction database to screen a new prescription. This is so critical that if for some reason you cannot get all your medicines filled at one pharmacy, be sure that each pharmacy you use has a complete list of all the medications you take. Here's an example of why this is important. One drug you take may go through an enzyme system in your liver where it is made inactive, but another drug you take may cause those liver enzymes to stop working. The result: the first drug does not become inactive but instead builds up to a toxic level in your bloodstream. Both doctors and pharmacists need to rely on computerized drug interaction databases to warn of potentially dangerous combinations.

Drug interactions are one concern. Another is that certain drugs can cause side effects in some people. It's important to know that side effects don't necessarily occur immediately. Sometimes a side effect will first appear months after you begin taking a drug.

Some people prefer to take all their heart medications at one time each day. But if you develop side effects, you might try spacing the medicines apart, taking an ACE inhibitor in the morning and a beta blocker in the evening, or vice versa. If that doesn't decrease the side effects, your doctor may lower the dose of one of the medicines.

The following risks and side effects are common for the standard drugs used in heart failure. (It is not a complete list. For a complete list, talk with your doctor or read the medication's package insert.) Most heart patients who are monitored carefully by their doctors don't develop serious side effects from their heart medications. If you experience any reaction or side effect, discuss it with your doctor before you stop taking a drug. If you develop a side effect that could be an emergency, stop taking the drug, call 911, and get yourself taken to a hospital.

ACE Inhibitors

The most common adverse effect is low blood pressure. ACE inhibitors were originally formulated to treat high blood pressure and are still used for that. But they are so beneficial in treating heart failure that they are used for this purpose even in people who have normal or naturally low blood pressure. So if you are on an ACE inhibitor, you must be monitored at regularly scheduled office visits to be sure your blood pressure does not get too low. Dizziness and feeling faint can be signs that your blood pressure is getting too low. To minimize side effects, most people are started on the lowest dose of an ACE inhibitor, and then slowly the dose is increased as tolerated. ACE inhibitors may cause low blood pressure and dizziness particularly when standing up from sitting or lying down. Getting up slowly can minimize this effect.

ACE inhibitors can also cause potassium buildup and kidney problems. These problems can be checked with a simple blood test, which should be done within 2 weeks after starting the medication. Kidney problems can be worsened by *nonsteroidal anti-inflammatory drugs* (NSAIDs) such as ibuprofen. Care must be used when NSAIDs and an ACE inhibitor are taken together, and blood should be checked relatively frequently. Anyone who has the condition called *bilateral renal artery stenosis* should absolutely not take an ACE inhibitor.

A dry cough is a relatively common side effect of ACE inhibitors. Cough is also a symptom of heart failure. Your doctor needs to know about your cough in order to determine what's causing it and how to proceed, so tell your doctor. Most people will get over a cough caused by the ACE inhibitor a couple of weeks after the drug is switched to an angiotensin receptor blocker.

A rare and potentially dangerous, even life-threatening, side effect of ACE inhibitors is swelling of the lips, tongue, gums, or throat. If you notice even the slightest swelling, stop taking the drug and have someone bring you to a hospital emergency room. Taking Benadryl or hydrocortisone may help relieve symptoms, but take these drugs only if your doctor says it's okay.

Angiotensin Receptor Blocker

An ARB has the effect of lowering blood pressure. It has many of the side effects of an ACE inhibitor but is thought to be better tolerated.

Beta Blockers

Beta blockers are started at low doses and slowly moved up to higher doses because going too quickly to a high dose can worsen the symptoms of heart failure. Like ACE inhibitors, beta blockers are used to treat high blood pressure, and common adverse effects are low blood pressure and a slowed heart rate. Either low blood pressure or a slow heart rate may cause dizziness and fainting. Carvedilol may lower blood pressure a little more than metoprolol succinate or bisoprolol.

Beta blockers may also cause fatigue. With time, this effect usually wears off. Heart failure can also cause fatigue. Report this symptom to your doctor to help sort out whether fatigue is a medication effect or a symptom of heart failure.

Men may develop erectile dysfunction, and women may have lower libido when taking beta blockers. Men who are taking a beta blocker and nitroglycerin *must not* take Viagra or similar drugs to correct their sexual dysfunction. Viagra and Viagra-like drugs increase the risk of low blood pressure, especially when taken with a nitrate, like nitroglycerin. This may be a problem if you develop chest pain with sexual activity and take nitroglycerin for relief. You could wind up in the emergency room. A number of men have done that.

Beta blockers may exacerbate fluid retention in a small percentage of people with unusually severe heart failure. In some people, beta blockers will cause detailed dreams, even nightmares. Exactly what happens in the brain to cause the dreaming is not understood.

Some people on beta blockers experience depression. In any particular person, it is not known for sure whether the drug or the heart failure is the cause. Regardless, the depression can be treated with sertraline, shown in the Sad Heart Trial to be a very safe drug in people with heart disease. People who have heart disease should avoid *tricyclic antidepressants* because they increase the risk of rhythm problems with the heart.

Loop Diuretics

Since diuretics cause frequent urination, they also cause the loss of potassium, magnesium, and sodium. For this reason, the major adverse effects of loop diuretics are dehydration and a decline in potassium and magnesium levels. If potassium drops too low, a deadly arrhythmia can be triggered in your heart. Use of potassium supplements or the drug spironolactone can help maintain blood potassium levels. An information sheet or a sticker on your medication bottle may suggest that you eat foods high in potassium while taking this medication. But ask your doctor before doing this. *Never take potassium supplements or deliberately eat foods high in potassium without the approval of your doctor.* Keep in mind that ACE inhibitors increase levels of potassium, which could cancel out the effect of another drug lowering your level of potassium; so if you are taking multiple drugs for heart failure, doctors need to monitor your blood periodically to be sure your potassium levels are in a normal range.

Dehydration can cause both low blood pressure and kidney failure. Severe heart failure may also cause low blood pressure and kidney failure. Based on a physical examination and your symptoms, your doctor will determine if you are dehydrated. Diuretics can also cause or worsen gout, a painful disorder of joints occurring commonly in fingers and toes.

Digoxin

Low-dose digoxin is usually very well tolerated. Nausea, vomiting, and loss of appetite are the first signs of digoxin toxicity. Other problems include palpitations and a slowed or irregular rhythm of the heartbeat. A level of digoxin that is too high can cause a potentially fatal heart rhythm. Digoxin may also cause vision problems and confusion. All of these side effects occur more frequently with higher doses.

Some drugs, such as amiodarone and spironolactone, may increase the level of digoxin in the blood. Amiodarone can cause these levels to increase dramatically. When these drugs are started in a person already taking digoxin, periodic blood tests are needed, and an adjustment of the digoxin dose is often required. People taking digoxin need to have healthy kidney function because the drug is excreted through the kidneys, and poor kidney function could mean stronger side effects.

DRUG INFORMATION FOR PEOPLE RECENTLY HOSPITALIZED WITH SEVERE HEART FAILURE

One diuretic that is not a loop diuretic and that has been shown to improve survival in people with severe heart failure is *spironolactone.* Spironolactone is recommended for people who have recurrent or severe symptoms of heart failure, often with frequent hospitalizations, despite the use of an ACE inhibitor, beta blocker, loop diuretic, and digoxin.

Potassium levels need to be watched carefully through blood tests because spironolactone may cause these levels to increase dramatically. Some deaths have resulted. Both men and women can get enlarged, painful breasts because spironolactone hits the estrogen receptor and the body thinks spironolactone is estrogen. It does not affect estrogen-fed cancers. A newer drug, eplerenone, works similarly but does not cause painful breast enlargement.

DRUG INFORMATION FOR PEOPLE HOSPITALIZED WITH ESPECIALLY SEVERE HEART FAILURE

When people are sick enough to be hospitalized with heart failure, a variety of drugs are administered to them for a short time, often intravenously, to get them better quickly. Doctors try to get patients off these drugs and onto more standard cardiac treatment as soon as possible, because some of these drugs cause lethal arrhythmias. More information on this subject can be found in chapter 15.

DRUGS TO AVOID OR USE WITH GREAT CARE IN CERTAIN POPULATIONS

People with heart failure are often elderly and have several other medical problems. Many take multiple medications for conditions other than heart failure, and some of these medications can interact with drugs taken for heart failure. What follows is a discussion of three of the most common conditions, the most common medications prescribed for them, and how these medications may interact with those taken by people with heart failure.

Diabetes

Metformin, used to control blood sugar in people with diabetes mellitus, is excreted from the body in urine and will tend to build up in the blood if the kidneys do not work well, which may be the case in people with heart failure. This buildup can lead to *lactic acidosis,* a life-threatening accumulation of acid lactate in the blood. Metformin, however, is an extremely important therapy in the treatment of diabetes. If you have diabetes and heart failure, you may need to take metformin, and in that case it must be monitored carefully by your physician.

Rosiglitazone and pioglitazone are newer drugs used in the management of diabetes. They may cause fluid retention in people prone to it, such as people with heart failure. The FDA has asked manufacturers to put the federal agency's strongest warning, a boxed warning, on these and all drugs in the category of *thiazolidinediones,* alerting consumers to a risk of developing or worsening heart failure. The warning also states that these drugs should not be used by people with serious or severe heart failure. People with heart failure should use these drugs *only* with careful follow-up with a doctor. Insulin may be an appropriate alternative to metformin and the glitazones, although insulin may also cause fluid retention.

Asthma

Many people with asthma do not have to avoid all beta blockers. A person whose asthma is under control or who occasionally uses a bronchodilator can take a beta blocker provided it is one such as metoprolol succinate, which blocks primarily the beta one receptor. Doctors are cautious about giving someone with asthma a beta blocker, because it can interfere with the ability of a common asthma rescue inhaler to work, and it can cause bronchospasm. Albuterol and other rescue inhalers that work like it relieve an asthma attack by contacting the beta two receptor. Two of the three beta blockers used in heart failure—carvedilol and bisoprolol—block both beta one and beta two receptors and therefore should be avoided by persons with severe asthma. At high enough doses, even metoprolol can block both beta one and beta two receptors, so doctors must regulate the dosage carefully, communicating with the patient and his asthma doctor. I find that metoprolol succinate can be safely taken by people except those with the most severe cases of asthma. Close follow-up with a physician is required when someone with asthma starts taking a beta blocker. People with *chronic obstructive pulmonary disease* (COPD) without asthma symptoms usually tolerate beta blockers.

Gout

Diuretics may cause gout, for which a common therapy is a nonsteroidal anti-inflammatory drug (NSAID) such as ibuprofen or naproxen. These drugs cause fluid retention through a direct effect on the kidney. Fluid retention will worsen the signs and symptoms of heart failure. In addition, NSAIDs may cause temporary kidney failure, which occurs more commonly in people with heart failure. NSAIDs and the newer *COX-2 inhibitor* celecoxib should be used carefully if at all by anyone with heart failure. Other COX-2 inhibitors, such as rofecoxib, have been withdrawn from the market because of dangerous side effects.

OTHER DRUGS TO AVOID OR USE WITH SPECIAL CARE

Certain *calcium channel blockers* lower blood pressure and decrease the strength of heart contraction. Because of this, they worsen heart failure in people with a low ejection fraction. The calcium channel blockers to be avoided if you have heart failure and a low ejection fraction are verapamil, diltiazem, and nifedipine.

A variety of drugs known as *antiarrhythmic drugs* used to control irregular heartbeats should not be taken by people with heart failure unless they have an implantable cardioverter defibrillator. Although these drugs are used to control arrhythmias, paradoxically they may also worsen arrhythmias, especially in people with heart failure. The drugs are quinidine, procainamide, mexiletine, encainide, flecainide, and propafenone. Amiodarone is probably the safest antiarrhythmic agent for people with heart failure if an antiarrhythmic drug is needed beyond beta blockers.

A CHANGING LANDSCAPE: TAILORING TREATMENT TO SPECIFIC POPULATIONS AND INDIVIDUALS

Gender and race are sometimes factors in how people respond to the medications used to treat heart failure. Women, non-Caucasians, children, and the elderly are often underrepresented in clinical trials, and therefore doctors do not know if our standard drug therapy for heart failure works in all population subgroups. This is an area of intensive research interest and will likely be worked out with time.

In 2004, a randomized trial of over 1,000 African Americans with heart failure taking either BiDil (a combination of the drugs isosorbide dinitrate and hydralazine) or a placebo was stopped early because BiDil was shown to have significant benefit over the placebo. The African American Heart Failure Trial (A-HeFT) was the first time a drug for heart failure was tested in a population composed only of African Americans. It is now widely used for African Americans who have heart failure.

In 2005 the Women's Health Study (WHS), a huge study of nearly 40,000 women over the age of 45, revealed that aspirin does not help prevent heart attacks in middle-aged women as it does in men, although aspirin does help prevent strokes in middle-aged women. After age 65, aspirin showed benefit against both heart attacks and strokes in women.

How best to prevent stroke is controversial. People with heart failure and a low ejection fraction appear to be at greater risk of a stroke caused by a blood clot breaking off from inside the heart and lodging in the brain. Some people are prescribed warfarin or aspirin to prevent such a stroke. There is no scientific evidence to prove which of these medications is more appropriate or even if any therapy is required at all.

Some cases are more clearly defined. People who should be taking warfarin are those in atrial fibrillation, with a clot in the heart visible on echocardiography, with a prior history of stroke, or with certain forms of valvular heart disease.

At some point, medicine will likely be able to predict who will respond to which drugs based on a genetic analysis obtained from a drop of blood. Exciting progress is being made in personalized medicine. For instance, knowing who has a variation of a gene associated with heart function can be crucial. In a 2008 study published in *Nature Medicine,* Stephen B. Liggett of the University of Maryland and researchers at Washington University found why some African Americans don't respond to beta blockers. They have their own. In a study of 375 African Americans, 40 percent had a variant of the *GRK5* gene that acted as a natural beta blocker, protecting against the need for a heart transplant or death from heart failure.

Chapter Review: Drugs to Take

- ***If you have a weakened heart muscle (systolic dysfunction) but no symptoms of heart failure:*** **ACE inhibitor and beta blocker.**
- ***If you have a weakened heart muscle (systolic dysfunction) with symptoms of heart failure:*** **Beta blocker, ACE inhibitor, loop diuretic, and possibly digoxin. If you were recently hospitalized for heart failure or are experiencing severe, limiting symptoms, add spironolactone or eplerenone.**
- ***If you have a normal heart contraction (nonsystolic heart failure):*** **Angiotensin receptor blocker (ARB), loop diuretic, and, in some cases, a beta blocker.**

To Take Charge

- **Know what medicines should work best for you and take them faithfully.**
- **Get all your prescriptions filled at one pharmacy so the computer can check for drug interactions.**
- **Report symptoms and side effects to your doctor, keeping in mind that a side effect may begin occurring months after you started taking a drug.**

6

Conversations of the Heart

Arrhythmias and Pacemakers

It is the iron man, always working. Powerful, indomitable, ignored, taken for granted. As long as your heart serves you well and faithfully, you are unaware of its chambers beating, its valves continually opening and closing like the gates of a dam, herding torrents of blood into narrow tunnels that spread throughout your body, pulse points authenticating the heart at work, at the ready for checking. But you never check. Why would you? You're not aware of your heart at work. It is the silent guardian, so quiet you don't notice it's there.

Until one day it talks to you.

Now, with a jolt, you do feel your heart. And it's unsettling. Something doesn't seem right. The beating seems too fast. Racing. So you stop to take your pulse, fingers on your wrist, and then in the midst of the staccato beats something more peculiar happens. Nothing. Your fingers are your stethoscope, and you keep listening to your heart. And there it is again. Nothing. A skipped heartbeat. And then the racing thump, thump, thump, thump is back. This is tachycardia, an *arrhythmia,* and with it a skipped beat. And just like that, your heart has your full attention.

There are many different types of irregular heartbeats. In all of them, your heart breaks its silence and lets you know that something is wrong. A heart beating too slowly produces *bradycardia,* making you feel sluggish and tired. A heart beating too fast causes *tachycardia,* and you feel the unsettling erratic nature of your heartbeat. Within each of these two broad categories are many subcategories. The most urgent malfunction of the heart's rhythm is *ventricular fibrillation,* when the heart screams to be noticed because it has begun shaking uncontrollably and is unable to right itself and begin pumping blood again. Fail to pay attention immediately and you will die. (The person this happens to will not have time to respond; someone who sees the person collapse must respond quickly. See chapter 7, "Straight Talk about Sudden Death.")

How much trouble you are in when your heart beats irregularly depends on what part of the heart is misfiring. *Atrial fibrillation,* a form of tachycardia, makes your heart feel like it's fluttering. It is scary but not always harmful. Atrial fibrillation can run in families, although the gene has not yet been identified.

Michael Conron first felt his heart in 1995 as he lay down for the night on his left side. He turned on his right side and no longer felt anything. Over a period of years, the distressing feeling occurred on and off when he lay down, and the financial officer had several tests to try to pinpoint the reason for the erratic heartbeat. It bothered him enough that he underwent cardioversion several times. In this 10-minute procedure, he was put into a twilight sleep, and his heart was given a jolt of electricity to restore its normal rhythm. But the heart can once again fall into an abnormally rapid beating problem, as Michael's did, which is why he again would go in for the electric shock to reset his heart.

Nothing serious has been discovered as a cause for his abnormal heartbeat, and he takes nadolol, a beta blocker, to slow the beat. In atrial fibrillation, the atria kind of wiggle rather than rhythmically contract. This motion can cause blood clots to develop, and they can break off and float away in the bloodstream, causing a stroke if they lodge in the brain and a pulmonary embolus if one lodges in the lung. So Michael also takes an anticoagulant, warfarin, to prevent blood clots. Today he still feels an erratic heartbeat occasionally, but he is no longer worried by it. His brother and a sister also have it, and he wonders if it is genetic.

NORMAL ELECTRICAL ACTIVITY

Every one of us has a pacemaker built into our hearts. The electrical activity that triggers the normal heartbeat begins in the right atrium, in the *sinoatrial node,* a tiny mass of muscle fibers the size and shape of an almond. This almond is the heart's natural pacemaker, which sets the pace of the heart at 60 to 100 beats per minute at rest. As you move around, the pacemaker triggers a faster heart rate to allow the heart to

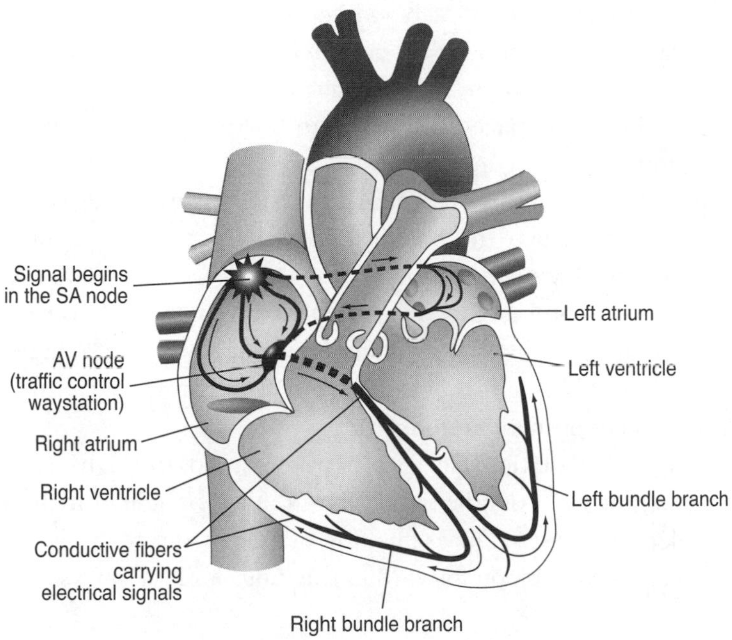

Electrical system in a normal heart

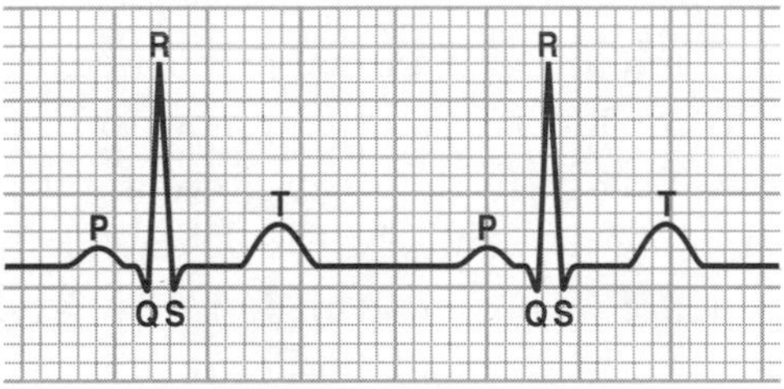

ECG of a normal heart rhythm

Figure 6.1. The normal electrical system of the heart. The pacemaker of the heart, the sinoatrial (SA) node, located in the right atrium, fires an electrical charge that spreads through both the left and right atria to the atrioventricular (AV) node. Here the pulse slows, allowing time for the atria to contract before the ventricles. From the AV node, the electrical wave spreads through special conductive fibers called the right and left bundle branch to activate the right and left ventricles. Atrial electrical activity, ventricular electrical activity, and the return to the baseline ventricular state cause the P wave, QRS complex, and the T wave, respectively.

pump an adequate amount of blood needed for the increased exertion. Exercising or playing sports will trigger the fastest heart rate. Getting frightened will also trigger a fast heart rate because the heart's pacemaker cranks up the pace in response to hormones the adrenal gland secretes under stress (figure 6.1).

From the pacemaker, the electrical activity passes through both the right and the left atria to the *atrioventricular node* (AV node), a peanut-sized waystation that slows conduction of the electrical impulse. The lag allows the atria to contract first, followed by the ventricles. This rhythmic contraction of first the atria and then the ventricles is critical in moving blood forward, because if they contracted at the same time, little or no blood would get pushed out to the body.

Leaving the waystation, electrical activity spreads through specialized heart tissue, the right bundle branch and the left bundle branch, which act like electrical wires. They signal the muscle of the ventricles to contract, which propels blood forward to the lungs and the body.

TOO SLOW, TOO FAST: HOW COME?

A heart can beat too slowly in many ways. The heart's pacemaker can become defective and fall behind with its electrical signals. The pacemaker may be fine and trigger a normal number of heartbeats, but the waystation, the AV node, may cause too much of a delay. When the waystation isn't working correctly, it can prevent some or all electrical activity from getting to the ventricle. Or the bundle branches can be defective. The result of any of these malfunctions is a heart that beats too slowly at rest and with exertion. Most commonly, these are intermittent slowdowns with stretches of normal electrical conduction producing normal heartbeats in between episodes.

A heart can also beat too fast in many ways. The heart's pacemaker can become defective and trigger heartbeats too quickly. New pacemakers will sometimes arise in the atria and take over the heartbeat at a rate that is too fast. Atrial flutter and atrial fibrillation are classic examples of what happens when areas of the atria run away with the heartbeat. *Atrial flutter* is a fairly regular beating because there are relatively few areas involved, while atrial fibrillation is chaotic because many areas are involved at the same time (figure 6.2). Think of atrial flutter as one person speak-

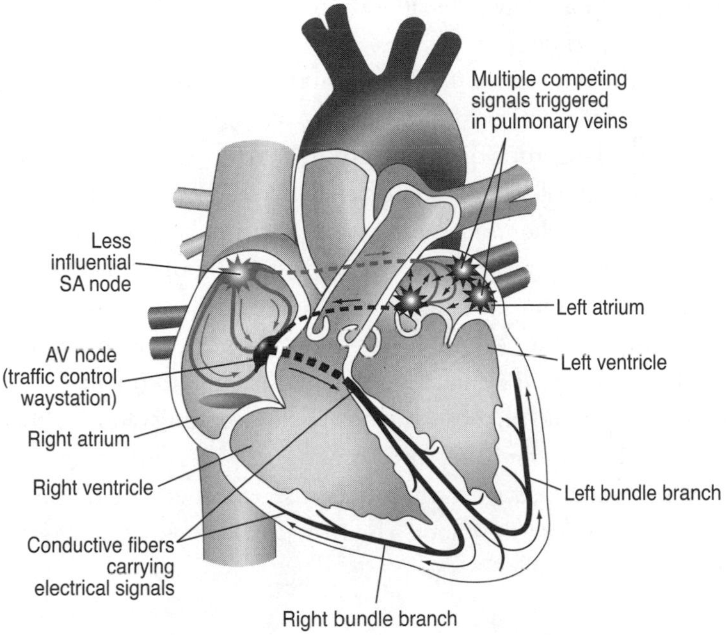

Electrical system in atrial fibrillation

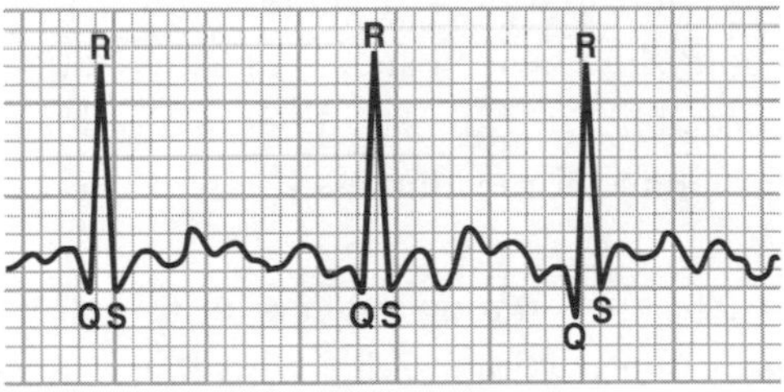

ECG of atrial fibrillation

Figure 6.2. Atrial fibrillation. Electrical activity in atrial fibrillation is often generated in the pulmonary veins. The SA node is suppressed because the electrical activity in the atria is much faster than in the SA node. This causes the absence of P waves and an irregular rhythm that show up on an ECG. Usually this rhythm is faster than normal, but at times it may be slower than normal.

ing very quickly, and atrial fibrillation as many people speaking quickly and at the same time.

Areas of the ventricles can also become abnormal pacemakers. When one or more areas are involved, this is *ventricular tachycardia* (figure 6.3). But the most dangerous of all irregular heartbeats is ventricular fibrillation. If atrial fibrillation is a chorus of people's voices talking or singing in different pitches and speeds, then ventricular fibrillation is a full orchestra warming up, with every instrument loudly blasting different notes at the same time. When this happens in the heart, the wildly fast, totally chaotic rhythm originates in many areas of the ventricle simultaneously, rendering the heart helpless (figure 6.4). Now just a shaking piece of flesh with no purpose, the heart stops sending blood and oxygen to the body. Unless the heart's person is wearing an implanted defibrillator, or someone can, within minutes, use external electric paddles to shock the heart back to a normal rhythm, the person dies. This is sudden death.

TRIGGERS FOR ARRHYTHMIAS

Arrhythmias may occur in a completely normal heart but are much more common in abnormal hearts. People who have heart failure are more prone to both slow heartbeats and fast, chaotic heartbeats than people with a normal heart. Abnormalities at a cellular level—scarring from a prior heart attack, for example—trigger the creation of arrhythmias.

Many medications are common triggers for arrhythmias. Whole Web sites are dedicated to discussing medications that can cause ventricular tachycardia based on the length of time it takes for the heart to recover from electrical excitation, a diagnosis known as the *long QT syndrome*. Your electrocardiogram will show if you have long QT syndrome. Although rare in the general population, it is common in people with heart failure. Antibiotics, decongestants, antidepressants, and most antiarrhythmics are a few categories of drugs that can cause arrhythmias in someone who has long QT syndrome. You can read more about drugs to be avoided by someone with this diagnosis at http://long-qt-syndrome.com.

Alcohol and recreational drugs can trigger a host of different arrhyth-

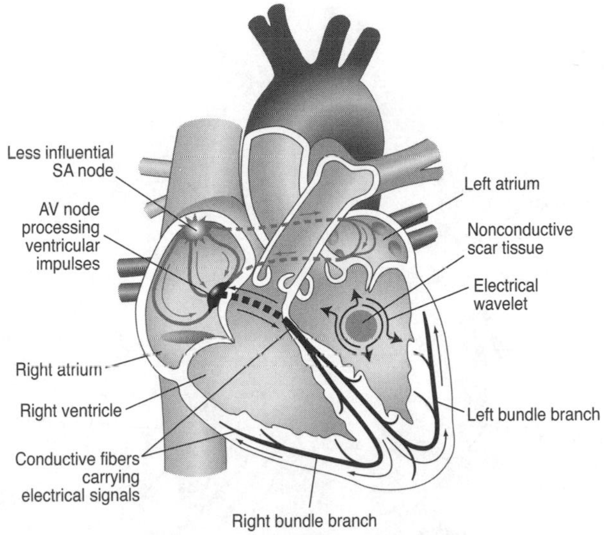

Electrical system in ventricular tachycardia

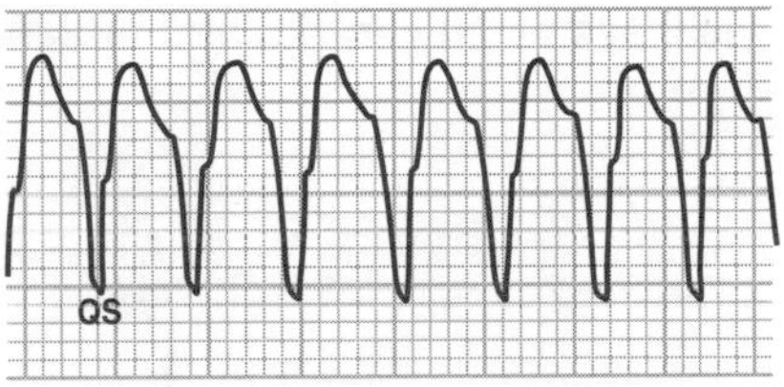

ECG of ventricular tachycardia

Figure 6.3. Ventricular tachycardia. Abnormal electrical pacemakers sometimes develop from cells or small groups of cells that have become loose cannons. Instead of accepting their electrical charge from the heart's normal pacemaker, they spark electrical activity that begins rolling around and around a glob of scar tissue that does not itself conduct electrical impulses. Normally the electrical charge would travel down the normal activation pathway until it gets to the scar and then go around the scar in both directions, meeting on the other side, where it would collide, joining again to stimulate the ventricle. But this time one of the electrical waves goes around the scar much more slowly, and when it gets to the other side, the faster wave has already gone by, so the electrical charge can then stimulate the muscle around the scar. The slower electrical wave goes round and round the scar much like a race car going around a track. Each time the electrical wave goes around the scar, it triggers activation of the ventricle. This occurs quickly because the distance around the scar is small. This circuit acts like a fraudulent pacemaker, replacing for the time being the heart's normal pacemaker, and can be persistent or stop just as suddenly as it started. This continual re-entry of electrical activity into muscle around a scar is how ventricular tachycardia actually occurs. The mechanism of atrial flutter is similar to this except that it occurs in atrial tissue and involves a larger circuit.

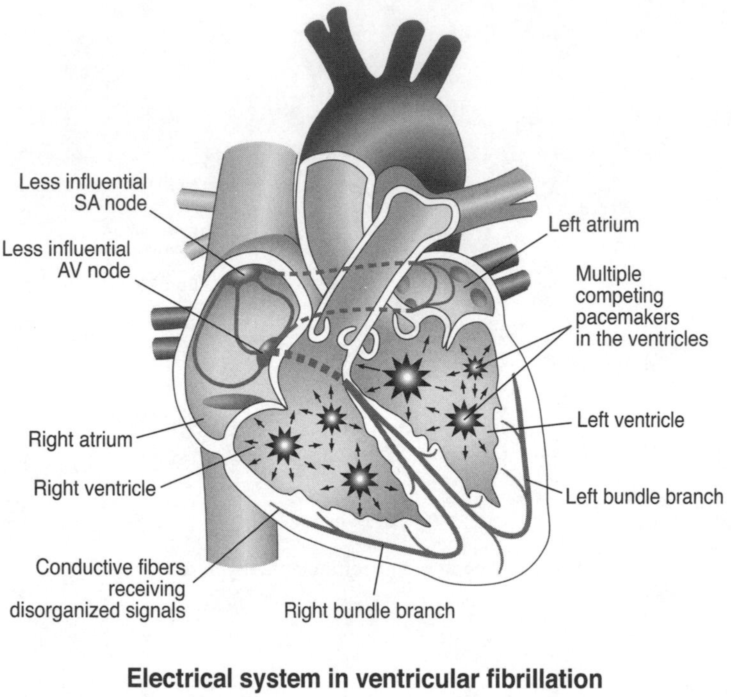

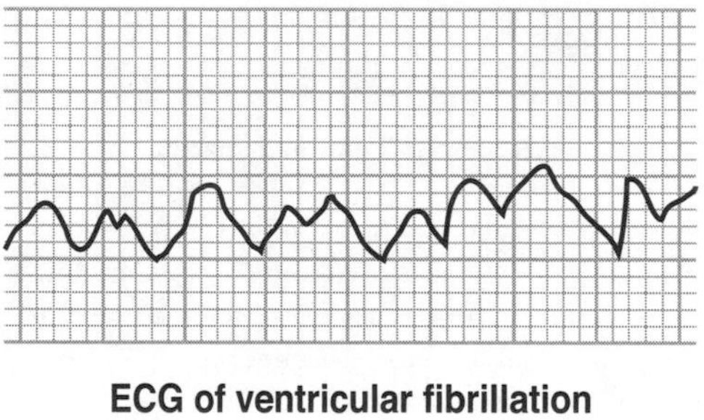

Figure 6.4. Ventricular fibrillation and sudden death. In ventricular fibrillation, total chaos ensues, with multiple ventricular pacemakers firing at once. This leads to ineffective pumping action and sudden death.

mias. Stress, caffeine, sleep deprivation, and sleep apnea are all common triggers for a variety of arrhythmias.

People usually describe them as a sense of fluttering in their chest, palpitations that start and stop abruptly. If the heart rate is very fast or very slow, fainting or dizzy spells can occur, the result of ineffective blood flow to the brain. Many people with a slow heart rate complain of fatigue or weakness that improves once their heart rate returns to normal.

COMMON ARRHYTHMIAS IN HEART FAILURE

Many people with atrial fibrillation also have atrial flutter. The symptoms are very similar to atrial fibrillation, and the treatment is the same, including warfarin to prevent blood clots and a beta blocker to keep the heart from beating too fast. Cardioversion is also performed, just as in atrial fibrillation. People who continue to be bothered by atrial flutter may want to consider a procedure called *ablation therapy*, which cures the problem 98 percent of the time. Electrophysiologists, cardiologists with special training in the care of people with arrhythmias, put wires into the heart to locate the part of the atrium that is participating in the atrial flutter. Then they use radiofrequency energy to burn that malfunctioning area. The procedure is sometimes used for atrial fibrillation, but it is less effective, achieving a cure about 70 percent of the time. The risks are low, with a 1 percent chance of something serious happening.

Ventricular tachycardia is much like atrial flutter only originating in the ventricles. Unlike atrial flutter, it will often lead to fainting and carries with it an ominous prognosis. The treatment is different. Medications may be used, but often a defibrillator is placed to prevent sudden death because ventricular tachycardia can quickly become ventricular fibrillation. And ventricular fibrillation quickly brings on loss of consciousness and sudden death.

Bradycardia is also common in heart failure. The symptoms that are associated with a heart rhythm that is too slow include lightheadedness, fainting, near fainting, and fatigue. Most bradycardias do not need to be treated with a pacemaker. Well-conditioned runners often have a slow resting heart rate that might be considered abnormal in other, less well-conditioned, people, and they certainly do not need a pacemaker. A medication such as a beta blocker may cause bradycardia as a side effect. The treatment then is to either stop the beta blocker or decrease the dose. In anyone with heart failure, stopping the beta blocker may not be a good option, because beta blockers improve survival in people with a weak heart muscle. For such people, the dose of the beta blocker is usually decreased, and a pacemaker is considered.

TREATING ABNORMAL HEART RHYTHMS

Treatment depends on the type of arrhythmia. Some are treated with drugs. Others require a pacemaker. Still others may require both drugs and a pacemaker. Treatment must be individualized.

Pacemakers

Pacemakers have evolved rapidly since their invention in the 1950s. A pacemaker basically consists of a battery to provide electrical stimulation and wires called leads that deliver the electrical stimulation to the heart when it is needed. The titanium unit, about the size of a silver dollar though much thicker, is implanted just under the skin in the upper left chest, and its leads run through veins to the heart. A pacemaker works by first sensing that electrical activity in the heart has been absent for a preset fraction of a second and then delivering an electrical signal that will cause the heart to contract. The pacemaker must also sense when the heart's own natural pacemaker resumes normal electrical activity so that the mechanical one only paces when it is needed. In some conditions, such as when a person has a weak heart muscle and left bundle branch block that delays electrical current on the left side of the left ventricle, the pacemaker typically is set to pace continually so that the left ventricle beats in sync.

Implanting a pacemaker normally takes a couple of hours and is done by an electrophysiologist in a cardiac catheterization lab. You will usually be unaware of your pacemaker, which works without causing any sensation. It is noticeable when you lie on your left side in bed and may cause a little soreness in your upper chest where it is placed, but most of the day you are not aware of it. A pacemaker may have one, two, or three leads. Each lead has the capability of sensing and pacing. The particular configuration of the leads depends on what the patient needs. The battery will need to be replaced every 5 to 10 years when it runs out of energy.

Pacemakers can be programmed to work in various ways and are individualized for each person depending on need. There are as many ways to set up a pacemaker as there are different types of heart rhythms. Be sure to discuss with your doctor the type of pacemaker you will get, see what one looks like, and ask about benefits and risks. The *biventricular pacemaker,* which is used to treat the symptoms of heart failure in people whose left ventricle is both weak and beating out of sync, is discussed below.

First, a word of caution about a right ventricular lead pacemaker. Some people who have a weak heart muscle and an unhealthy underlying conduction system can develop an artificial left bundle branch block if they use a right ventricular lead pacemaker. In this situation, pacing by a right ventricular lead creates an artificial left bundle branch block because electrical stimulation, starting at the tip of the lead in the right ventricle, spreads across the heart and hits one side of the left ventricle before it hits the other. Almost everyone with heart failure and a weak heart muscle should avoid pacing from only a right ventricular lead. If you have such a one-lead or two-lead pacemaker already, ask your cardiologist about having it replaced with a biventricular pacemaker. This is very important. Be sure you know what kind of pacemaker a doctor wants to put into you before you allow the procedure. Most electrophysiologists are switching to a biventricular system to help such patients.

Biventricular Pacemaker

Who can benefit from this type of pacemaker? Eligible patients have symptoms of heart failure and are on a good medical regimen, including an ACE inhibitor, a beta blocker and a loop diuretic. Someone with a weak heart muscle as evidenced by an ejection fraction of 30 percent or less and left bundle branch block will likely benefit from biventricular pacing, also known as *resynchronization therapy.* Biventricular pacing is done to resynchronize a left ventricle that no longer contracts all at the same time.

How does it work? In biventricular pacing, there are three leads—one in the right atrium, one in the right ventricle, and one placed as close to the left wall of the left ventricle as it can go. The two ventricular leads together restore a coordinated contraction to the left ventricle. (See figure 6.5.)

This is particularly important in left bundle branch block. Normally, from the AV node, electrical activity spreads to the ventricles through the right and left bundle branches. Think of these as wires. Electrical activity goes down both bundles at the same speed and so arrives at both

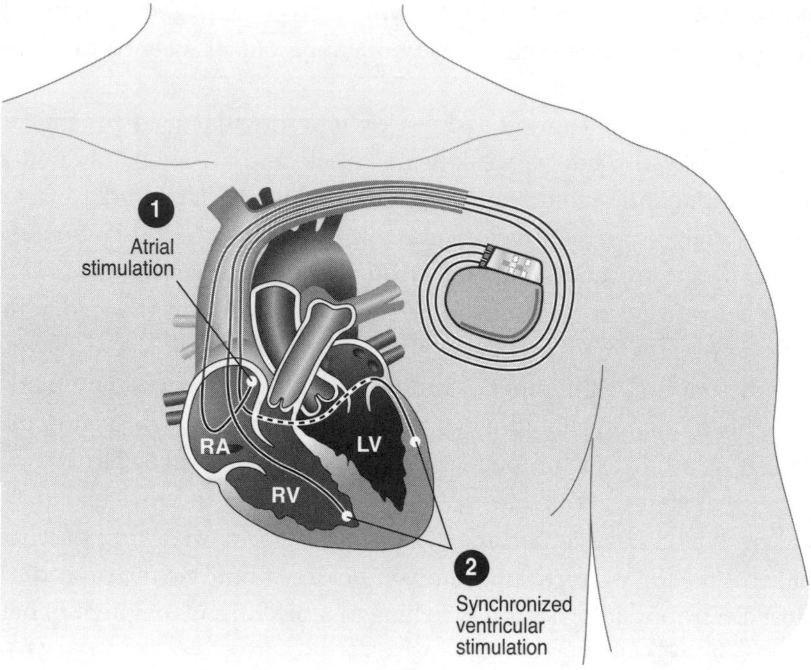

Figure 6.5. Biventricular pacemaker. The generator is usually located underneath the skin of the upper left chest. Wires, or leads, bring the electrical impulse to the heart itself. In a biventricular pacemaker, leads on the right and left sides of the left ventricle fire simultaneously, correcting a left ventricle that was beating out of sync.

sides of the left ventricle at the same time. In left bundle branch block, conduction of the electrical impulse is slowed down as it travels down the left bundle, and as a result the right wall of the left ventricle contracts ahead of the left wall. This is an inefficient way for the heart to beat and is an abnormality that many people with dilated cardiomyopathy have, for reasons we don't know.

Pacing both sides of the left ventricle at the same time with a biventricular pacemaker improves the strength of left ventricle contraction and causes the ventricle to contract as one unit because now the pacing bypasses the left bundle branch block. Studies show that biventricular pacing improves symptoms of heart failure and improves survival. Defibrillator function can be combined into the same device to further increase survival rates for people with heart failure and a weak heart. This combined device is a biventricular implantable cardiac defibrillator, or BiV-ICD. (Cardiac defibrillators are discussed in chapter 7.) A BiV-ICD, or a simple ICD that does not include a biventricular pacemaker, recognizes a lethal cardiac rhythm like ventricular fibrillation and delivers a shock to reset the heart to a normal rhythm. It can be a life-saving device.

A Caution to Heart Failure Patients about Other Types of Pacemakers

We want to emphasize that there are different types of pacemakers. Become informed about them. It is worth repeating that single-lead and dual chamber pacemakers that have leads attached only to the right ventricle or the right atria and right ventricle cause a disjointed contraction of the left ventricle as the electrical charge spreads across the heart, first to one part of the left ventricle and then to another. This may cause a pacemaker-induced type of left bundle branch block, or worse, an increase in heart failure symptoms in people with a weak heart muscle. Biventricular pacing, with its third lead attached to the left ventricle, eliminates this problem.

While many people in the general population in need of a pacemaker do not need biventricular pacing, those with heart failure and a weak left ventricle who need a pacemaker should strongly consider a biventricular pacemaker rather than one with only a right ventricular lead. Ask your doctor about biventricular pacing if you have heart failure and a weak heart muscle and are told you need a pacemaker.

Possible Pacemaker Problems

What are the potential problems? It may be impossible to get the left ventricular lead where it is most needed, way out on the left side of the left ventricle. If that is the case, the person will not benefit from biventricular pacing. Whether the left ventricular lead can be placed where it is most needed depends on the person's anatomy. Some people do not have an appropriately placed cardiac vein through which the left ventricular lead is normally placed. In such rare cases, a lead may be sewn directly on the outside of the left wall of the left ventricle during a brief operation using an incision made between the ribs. This procedure produces two scars, one over the pacemaker itself and the other between the ribs near the left breast.

Other problems can occur with a pacemaker. It might get infected, which is a disaster often requiring removal of the device. Rarely, the pacemaker and leads are defective and could need to be replaced or adjusted. The battery needs to be replaced every 5 to 10 years. The pacemaker or the leads might erode through the skin, though this occurs rarely, on the order of 1 in 1,000 cases. Breaking through the skin is more of a problem in skinny people.

Medications

For people with a weak heart muscle, most drugs used to treat rhythm disturbances are a real problem and should be avoided except in certain circumstances. As noted earlier, many of these drugs, called *antiarrhythmic* drugs, prolong the QT interval and cause an increase in ventricular tachycardia and sudden death—obviously an unwanted effect of a drug used to prevent rhythm disturbances.

This is not the case for all antiarrhythmic drugs. One of the beneficial properties of beta blockers is that they slow the heart rate and decrease the likelihood of ventricular tachycardia and sudden death. They do not prolong the QT interval, so they are not only safe to use in heart failure but are, in fact, a cornerstone of therapy. Beta blockers are also used to slow the heart rate in people with atrial flutter, atrial fibrillation, and certain other, less common, fast atrial rhythms.

Calcium channel blockers such as diltiazem are prescribed for the same purpose. Unfortunately, diltiazem is not a good drug to use in people with a weak heart muscle, because it further depresses the strength of left ventricular contraction and increases the symptoms of heart failure. Sometimes this drug is given intravenously to a patient to abruptly slow a fast heart rate, but it is not generally used as a long-term drug in patients with a weak heart muscle.

There are a host of other antiarrhythmic drugs, all of which have been shown to increase death, especially in people with a weak heart muscle who are prone to the effects of QT prolongation. Examples include procainamide, mexiletine, flecainide, sotalol, and quinidine.

Other than beta blockers, the only other usable antiarrhythmic is amiodarone, which rarely prolongs the QT interval and in several large studies has shown no effect on mortality in people with a weak heart muscle. Besides beta blockers, amiodarone currently may be the most effective antiarrhythmic drug. In atrial flutter and atrial fibrillation, it is used to slow the heart rate and prevent recurrence. Unfortunately, amiodarone has several serious side effects that limit its use, including problems with the liver, lung, and thyroid. It must be taken in the lowest dose that works and with careful monitoring by a cardiologist.

In some specific instances, antiarrhythmic drugs other than beta blockers or amiodarone may be taken by people with a weak heart muscle. For instance, people who have a defibrillator that repeatedly goes off for ventricular tachycardia may be started on amiodarone to decrease the number of times they will need to get a shock from the defibrillator. If a person has a serious side effect from amiodarone, she may be switched to another drug, such as sotalol, which most physicians would not be willing to prescribe to a person with a weak heart muscle without the backup of a defibrillator. This is a rare situation.

Whatever awakening you have experienced with your heart, one thing is for sure. Once you've engaged in a conversation with your heart, you feel an appreciation for it you didn't have before. We hope that any future conversations you have will be whispers and not shouts.

7

Straight Talk about Sudden Death

Should I Get an Implantable Cardioverter Defibrillator?

Many people diagnosed with heart failure will not die from it. But there are two ways that some people will. One is that the heart failure progressively gets worse over a period of years, or gets better for a while and then gets worse, eventually leading to death from heart failure. The other is sudden cardiac death. In this chapter, we will talk directly to you about sudden death, because the more you know, the better prepared you will be to try to prevent this intruder from cutting your life short. And that's the scary part about sudden death—not the way you die, but that it can happen way too early in someone's life and happen quickly, with no warning and only minutes to get help.

There is much outdated information on the Internet and in various publications about the rate of death in heart failure overall and the rate of sudden death from heart failure. We don't think there are accurate figures available on present-day heart failure death rates that reflect the growth in the use of such life-prolonging treatments as beta blockers, ACE inhibitors, implantable cardioverter defibrillators (ICDs), and heart transplants. We can only offer some glimpses into statistics on sudden death.

We know from one five-year study of patients with mild to moderate heart failure and a weakened heart muscle that only about 5 percent per year of the 829 patients with an ICD had an appropriate shock. If we assume that an appropriate shock represents an averted episode of sudden cardiac death, than the rate of sudden death in similar patients without an implanted defibrillator would be 5 percent per year.

Another study at Brigham and Women's Hospital in Boston, Massachusetts, found that 21 percent of patients with advanced heart failure experienced sudden death. This retrospective study examined the records of 160 patients who died of heart failure between January 2000 and October 2003. Far more common, the doctors found, was that people die of heart failure after a long course that frequently leads to kidney insufficiency in the last six months before death. These patients typically have many hospitalizations and die of complications of heart failure and not sudden death.

Although this Harvard-affiliated hospital study offers a small window into how heart failure patients die in the twenty-first century, we need a much larger and more inclusive study to really understand how people with heart failure die in this era. This prospective study would need to enroll thousands of people diagnosed with heart failure, ranging from those who feel well and are working at their jobs to those who are homebound or in hospitals experiencing severe symptoms. Participants should include the patients of community doctors as well as those seen at major medical centers. Only then can patients, families, and doctors find out what the overall rate of death from heart failure is and what the rate of sudden death is.

In general, we can say that in people who are being treated for heart failure, survival decreases as symptoms of heart failure increase. People with severe symptoms of heart failure, despite appropriate medical therapy, are more likely to die of their condition than of sudden death. Those with few symptoms are much less likely to die, but if they do die, it is more likely to be sudden.

This possibility of sudden death separates heart failure from most other illnesses or conditions. You may go through a period after your diagnosis when you feel you are living on edge, that life itself is uncertain. It's natural for anyone diagnosed with heart failure to feel scared of dying suddenly, without warning. Those close to you will be just as worried as you are about this risk. You may want to talk with a cardiologist about whether you are a candidate for an ICD, which is placed under the skin in your chest and attached to your heart. It can sense a lethal heart rhythm, correct it, and prevent sudden death. It does not prevent death from anything other than an electrical problem that turns into a lethal arrhythmia. In chapter 6 we described how one version of the ICD, the BiV-ICD, works. Later in this chapter, we discuss the rewards and risks of having an ICD.

A PERSONAL NOTE

First, though, I (Mary) want to share with you that there is a good side to sudden death. Having experienced that part of sudden death that the person dying is aware of, I can suggest to you that sudden cardiac death is probably the most pleasant way to leave this world. I developed a fatal heart arrhythmia during an angiogram. I was awake for the procedure and was not in any discomfort, and then a technician called out "Mary, how do you feel?"

"I feel strange," I responded. I had no pain and was not gasping for breath, but at that moment I realized my heart felt odd. It was out of sync, fibrillating. "Really strange." That was the last moment I was aware of. I was gone.

Luckily for me, the defibrillators were at hand, and I received four shocks to my heart before it started beating again. I did not feel or hear a thing and was amazed to learn, when I woke up, that I had been shocked with electric paddles on my chest and ribs, leaving temporary burn marks.

I had not had a heart attack. In fact, the angiogram would show that I had no blocked arteries. A heart attack happens when a cholesterol plaque buildup in an artery ruptures, blocking blood flow to a portion of the heart. A heart attack causes very uncomfortable symptoms, for men often a heavy pressure in the chest and pain radiating down the left arm, and for women nausea and fatigue. Many people have time to get to a hospital for treatment following a heart attack, though some will collapse and die if their heart is so affected that it develops a wild arrhythmia and cannot beat.

But people with heart failure who die suddenly usually do not have a heart attack. They can be feeling fine one minute, and the next, their heart goes into ventricular fibrillation. They may have time to feel as I did that something is wrong with their heart as it begins to shake instead of beat. Then almost immediately they are unconscious. If they are not wearing a defibrillator, and if no one can reach them within minutes with electric paddles to shock their heart back to a normal beating pattern, brain death will begin and shortly become irreversible.

I am so glad I was resuscitated, because there's much I have to live for and want to accomplish. But when my time comes, at an age when I feel I've accomplished most everything I can, if I could pick the way I will die, it would definitely be sudden cardiac death. I can honestly say I recommend it. And dying this way would not frighten me at all.

The good thing about sudden death, the only good thing, is the absence of misery. So, while your family and friends will experience the shock and the loss of your leaving, they can take comfort in knowing that you did not suffer. And that's a big thing for you and for them.

How you view sudden death may depend more on when it happens in your life or in the life of a loved one—at what age and in what state of health—rather than that it happens suddenly.

NEAR DEATH EXPERIENCE

A curious phenomenon associated with cardiac arrest is the "near death" experience. Between 10 and 20 percent of people who have survived an episode of sudden cardiac death describe one or more of the following features occurring while they were technically dead: hearing the news of their death from doctors or their family; a feeling of peace; sound described as beautiful music, ringing, or buzzing; a tunnel; a sensation of being out of their body, sometimes associated with a sense of floating above and watching their body; meeting deceased friends or religious beings; being in the presence of a beautiful light or loving being; undergoing a life review; and making a decision to come back. We may never know what this means, and it may be nothing more than the effects of oxygen starvation on brain cells. It is interesting, nonetheless. Many people who have had this experience are reluctant to speak about it for fear of ridicule. Others view it as a religious experience and want to tell the world. The literature suggests it occurs more frequently than one might expect.

WHAT TRIGGERS SUDDEN DEATH?

Many different problems can lead to fatal heart rhythms. First, there is often a predisposition caused by any one of various genetic mutations. If a person has the right mutation and takes certain medications, the combination triggers the long QT syndrome discussed in chapter 6, in which the heart takes longer than normal to recover from electrical stimulation and goes into ventricular fibrillation.

Always discuss new medications and herbal supplements with your doctor, especially if you have a weakened heart muscle. Cocaine also causes sudden death.

Second, there are physical problems in the heart. These include the stress put on the heart by heart failure and the abnormalities that are a part of this condition, including a weakened heart, a heart not filling properly, valve problems, electrical wiring problems such as a left bundle branch block, a history of heart attack, and coronary artery disease. These stressors lead to changes in the structure of the heart itself. Sudden death in heart failure occurs more frequently in people who have had a recent fainting episode without a known explanation. People who have palpitations, the sense that their heart is racing or skipping beats, are also at higher risk.

Problems outside the heart can help trigger a lethal heart rhythm. An example is a serum potassium level that is too low. Stress, in general, plays a role. Recent major life changes such as the death of a spouse, or a major stressful event such as an earthquake, are associated with an increased risk of sudden death. Time of day can also play a role. Sudden death is more common in the early morning hours, especially on Monday mornings because of the stress of returning to work. It is more common in people with heart failure and sleep apnea, which is a disorder of sleep in which people periodically stop breathing for a short period many times a night. Sleep apnea is associated with loud snoring.

Triggers of sudden death are an area of much research. If doctors could reliably identify the triggers and help their patients avoid them, they surely would decrease the risk of sudden cardiac death.

HOW THE HEART LOSES CONTROL OF ITS BEAT

Normal electrical activity that produces a heartbeat begins in the right atrium in the upper righthand side of the heart and then spreads across both atria and downward to the atrioventricular node (AV node), a small hump the size of a peanut, which separates the atria from the two lower chambers, the ventricles. The AV node acts as a speed bump to slow the travel of electricity. This delay allows the electrical activity to trigger contraction of first the atria and then the ventricles in a rhythmic and coordinated fashion.

Our hearts normally beat about 60 to 100 times a minute at rest. When the heart loses its normal beat, it is in an arrhythmia. Most arrhythmias are not life threatening. In fact, we get a fast heartbeat, or tachycardia (a heartbeat faster than 100 times a minute), every time we exercise. But normally during exercise, the heart does not actually lose control. It is called on to work harder and beat faster, and it does. Then it returns to its normal pace.

Very differently, a series of events can cause the heart to misfire, then lose its rhythm altogether, and quickly go from being an essential part of a person to no part of the person. The potentially fatal problem begins when abnormally fast heartbeats don't originate where they are supposed to, in the top part of the heart, but instead originate in the lower heart in one of the ventricles. When the heart beats so quickly, it is unable to send enough blood to the brain, and the person may nearly faint or actually pass out. This ventricular tachycardia quickly can turn into ventricular fibrillation. The ventricles start shaking, the valves of the heart don't open and close to let the blood pass through, and even if they did, the heart is not generating enough pressure to move the blood out. Ventricular fibrillation is complete chaos and is not compatible with life. With no force to move blood flow to the brain, irreversible brain damage usually begins within 4 to 6 minutes, and brain death occurs shortly thereafter. Most sudden death results from ventricular tachycardia that quickly degenerates into ventricular fibrillation.

WHAT TO DO IF SOMEONE COLLAPSES

Every minute counts in saving the life of a person whose heart has stopped working. For every minute that goes by without a shock to restore the normal heartbeat, the chance for surviving sudden cardiac death decreases by about 10 percent. If someone with heart failure suddenly collapses, don't waste time hovering over the person, yelling and asking if she is okay and trying to get her to speak to you. She is not okay, and she is not going to speak to you until someone shocks her heart into beating again. Call 911 immediately to summon a paramedic, who will use electric paddles on the unconscious person's chest and ribs to shock the heart back into a normal rhythm. Begin cardiopulmonary resuscitation (CPR) while waiting for a defibrillator to arrive. If you live with someone with heart disease, you should take a CPR course to learn what to do in the event of sudden cardiac death.

Automatic external defibrillators designed for use by anybody are now located in airports, stadiums, and some other buildings. They are placed in crowded locations so that bystanders can give a shock while waiting for paramedics to arrive. The automatic external defibrillators will talk to you and tell you how to decide whether a shock needs to be delivered or not. Then they will talk you through how to use the device on an unconscious person. By using one, you may save a life!

WHAT CAN I DO TO REDUCE THE RISK OF SUDDEN DEATH?

There are things you can do to decrease your risk of sudden death, starting with medications. Some of the medications used to treat heart failure, such as beta blockers, ACE inhibitors, angiotensin receptor blockers, spironolactone, and aspirin, may decrease the risk of sudden cardiac death, but they do not eliminate it.

Lifestyle changes can be beneficial, too. Avoid smoking and illicit drug use. If you drink, limit alcoholic beverages to no more than one to two glasses per day. Reducing stress is important. Avoid it as much as possible and counteract it with exercise and finding things to laugh about and enjoy every day.

DEFIBRILLATOR THERAPY

The only sure way (99 percent sure) to prevent sudden death from heart failure is to wear an implantable cardioverter defibrillator (ICD). Made of inert titanium metal and powered by long-acting batteries, it is the size and thickness of a small cell phone and is placed just beneath the skin, usually in the left shoulder area. Wires run from the ICD metal base through a vein to your heart. The ICD monitors your heart for the development of ventricular tachycardia or ventricular fibrillation and

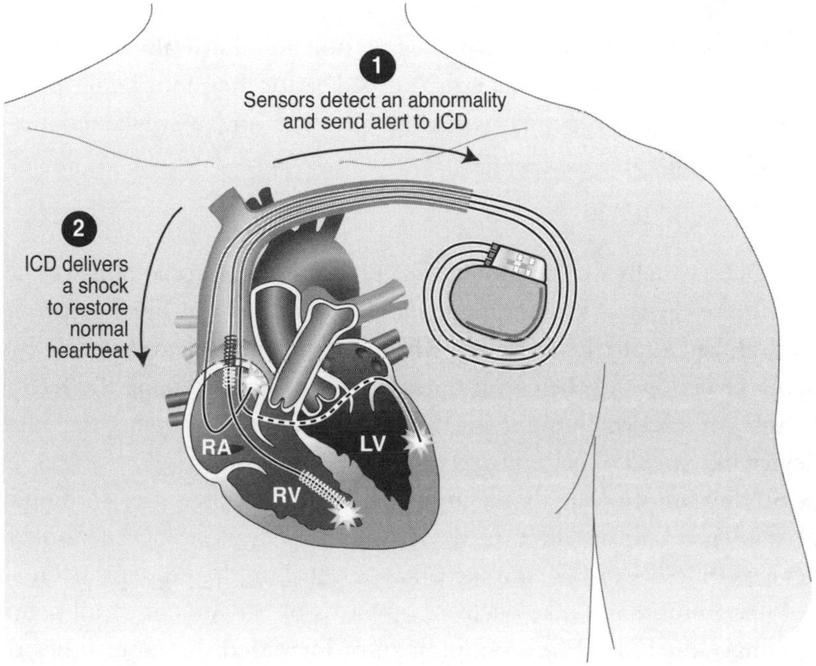

Figure 7.1. Implantable cardioverter defibrillator (combined with a biventricular pacemaker), also known as a BiV-ICD. If (1) sensors detect either ventricular tachycardia or ventricular fibrillation, (2) small coils located in two places on the right ventricular lead allow the ICD to shock the heart back into a normal rhythm. Biventricular pacing also occurs as shown in figure 6.5.

delivers a shock to restore your normal heartbeat within seconds of detecting an abnormality (figure 7.1).

If you are considering getting an ICD, ask your doctor to show you one and explain it to you so that you know what it looks like and how it works. Ask about risks and benefits.

The Benefits of ICDs

Modern ICDs also have a pacemaker function, so they will prevent your heart from beating too slowly. ICDs are 99 percent effective in preventing sudden cardiac death. In multiple clinical trials, ICDs have been shown to prolong the life of people who have suffered from one episode of sudden cardiac death already and survived. In addition, ICDs have been shown to prolong life in people with a low ejection fraction and symptoms of heart failure, whether or not they have already suffered an episode of sudden cardiac death. ICDs are therefore being placed in more and more people with heart failure and a weakened heart muscle.

The Risks of ICDs

An ICD is usually well tolerated, but there are some problems associated with these devices. For one, they have been known to fire inappropriately. This is not trivial. People who have been shocked describe it as being kicked in the chest by a horse. There is no mistaking the feeling. Rarely, an ICD will become infected, and when this happens, the entire device may need to be removed to cure the infection.

Studies are showing that a large number of people suffer continuing psychological distress after the device goes off. Stress, anxiety, fear of the device going off or failing to go off when it should, and depression are not uncommon and may occur in upwards of 30 percent of all people who have an ICD. These symptoms are increased the more times the device fires, especially if it fires many times in a row. One study found that people who wore an ICD mistakenly thought it protected them in far more cases than it does. The defibrillator only protects against death from a chaotic heart rhythm. It does not prevent heart attacks or dying from any other cause, such as a traumatic accident or cancer.

There is about a 1 percent risk of a complication during the procedure to implant an ICD. The risk of stroke, heart attack, or death during the procedure is actually much smaller, about one in several thousand. Expect the battery to last about 5 to 8 years; it will then need to be replaced. This is less time than a battery used in a pacemaker lasts because here a battery is asked to perform a different task—defibrillation—as well as pacing the heart when needed. There are rare recalls, only some of which require replacement of the device. However, it's not rare when it happens to you. I wear an ICD that was recalled after just a year, and my electrophysiologist called and told me to come in and get mine replaced.

The biggest problem of all with an ICD is that a doctor cannot tell most of us if we would definitely benefit from having one put in. A cardiologist can tell only those people who have suffered and survived an episode of sudden death that they should have and could clearly expect to benefit from an ICD. Otherwise, while the prevention of sudden death with an ICD in someone with a weak heart and symptoms of heart failure has been demonstrated in several clinical research studies, your doctor has limited abilities to predict if you personally will be one of the relative few who would otherwise suffer sudden death and therefore would benefit from an ICD.

Talk all this over with your doctor to make sure you understand the risks versus benefits before having an ICD implanted.

If you have an ICD and it fires, either appropriately or inappropriately, you may mistakenly believe that you will avoid future shocks by avoiding the particular activity you think caused the ICD to fire previously. By doing so, you may avoid activities that were enjoyable, such as sexual relations or modest exercise. Participating in a structured exercise rehabilitation program may actually help you resume normal activities. Some people find the unpredictable nature of firings unacceptable and avoid situations where receiving a shock might be embarrassing, such as at the theater or a party. You may be more likely to have these concerns if you had your ICD placed before you suffered an episode of sudden cardiac death. Some people find its presence comforting.

Participating in certain occupations, such as airline pilot, is restricted following implantation of an ICD. However, the vast majority of occupations will not be limited.

Many people wear an ICD that never fires and they go about their work and personal lives as though the device were not there. But for people whose ICD has fired multiple times and whose heart failure symptoms are severe, their spouse and other family members may be affected as well and assume a greater role in the running of daily family life. Such issues may result in feelings of anger and frustration in the person with heart failure or in their family. If you suffer from these problems, you and your family may find that taking part in an ICD support group is helpful. Make sure you all have a plan if the device goes off several times in a row. Know whom to contact should this occur. Try not to let the technology run your life. The ICD is there as a safety net. Don't let it become a trap that prevents you from doing things you enjoy (within reason, that is: you should reconsider that plan to go bungee jumping).

Nearly all the time, you will not be aware of your ICD. You can feel it when you turn over on your left side in bed, but such pressure will likely not affect the working of the ICD. If you accidentally fall, you will probably put out your hands to absorb some of the fall, and your ICD will usually not be affected. But you don't want anyone to press hard on it, especially if you are wearing a combination ICD-pacemaker known as a BiV-ICD, because that action could reset the pacemaker and affect its ability to direct the beating of your heart or to reset the heart's own pacing if it becomes too slow. Instructions should come with your ICD explaining what you need to avoid. You will not be able to have an MRI, for example, because you must keep your distance from strong magnets.

Keep in mind what an ICD does and does not do. Something Harvard cardiologist Akshay S. Desai, M.D., said in the December 15, 2004, issue of the *Journal of the American Medical Association* caught our eye because it is simply put: "ICD implantation, while effective in reducing sudden cardiac death, does not forestall the progression of heart failure." Desai, of Brigham and Women's Hospital in Boston, the principal investigator in a meta-analysis of ICD studies reported in the journal, makes an important point. In some people, heart failure will progress despite treatments. If you should reach a point where treatments are not working, and you are not a candidate for a heart transplant, or if you become ill with some other disease and reach a point where there are no more treatments, you may want to ask your cardiologist to turn off your ICD. At the end of life, you may appropriately decide you do not wish to be shocked. An ICD can always be turned off so that it is no longer capable of delivering a shock to your heart.

Most people with ICDs will lead active and happy personal and professional lives. As you consider an ICD, make sure you understand your risks and the potential benefits of the proposed therapy. Are there alternatives? What are the benefits and risks of the alternatives? What is your risk of doing nothing? Your doctor should be willing to take the time to discuss all this with you. The decisions you will be called on to make are difficult. Learn as much as you can about the benefits and problems of ICDs. Make a decision and go forward from there.

8

Surgical Treatments

There are times when medical therapy is not enough, and surgery may offer the chance to both improve symptoms and prolong life. Surgery has greater risk, so the benefits associated with surgery must also be greater. Ask your cardiologist what your alternatives are. The choice of what type of surgery and when it should be performed is not always easy. The choice of surgeon and hospital is critical to how well you will do. Look for a surgeon who routinely performs the operation you need. Then don't feel shy about asking questions, including these:

- How many of these operations have you performed?
- How many have you performed in the last year, and what is your success rate?
- What kinds of things have gone wrong when you did this surgery?
- Will you perform my surgery or will a resident or fellow or other doctor do part of it? If a doctor in training will handle part of my operation, will you be there the whole time to supervise?
- Given my condition and age and other medical problems, what do you believe will be the outcome of my surgery and my recovery?
- Do you believe I can safely undergo anesthesia?
- Will you make up a checklist of basic safety measures, and will my surgeons, anesthesiologist, nurses, and others assisting take time out to go over the checklist?

Each surgery discussed in this chapter—coronary artery bypass surgery, valve surgery, ventricular restoration, and passive restraint—should be used only in certain situations where other treatment would not be as effective. If your health allows you the time, always seek a second opinion from another cardiologist and another cardiac surgeon at a second hospital before agreeing to the surgery.

CORONARY ARTERY BYPASS SURGERY

Blood is constantly filling the heart, flowing through its four chambers, and rushing out to make its trip around the body and back. But all that blood circulating inside the heart does not provide what the heart itself needs to function. The heart's own blood supply comes from the coronary arteries. There are two main coronary arteries, the left and the right. The left coronary artery comes off the aorta just above the aortic valve. Very soon it splits into the left anterior descending coronary artery, which runs down the front of the heart, and the circumflex coronary artery, which wraps around the left side. The right coronary artery comes off the aorta just above the aortic valve and runs around the right side of the heart, often extending to the part closest to the diaphragm, a wide muscle separating the chest from the abdomen. Each coronary artery has many branches (see figure 1.3).

The threat to coronary arteries and the heart comes from a rupture of cholesterol plaque, which causes a blood clot. The clot plugs the artery, halting flow of blood beyond the clot and preventing nourishing blood from getting to the heart muscle. Without immediate treatment to open or bypass the blockage, a heart attack occurs, and the part of the heart that is starved of blood begins to die. Blockages in the left main coronary artery frequently cause major problems because so much of the heart depends on this artery for blood flow.

Less-than-complete cholesterol blockages also occur. When a plaque is large enough to block 70 percent of the artery, your heart usually lets you know there's a problem. Just as your legs can get very heavy and achy after you've run some distance, the part of your heart that is being deprived of oxygen screams for help. The heart's SOS is angina, an oppressive feeling in the middle of the chest that often moves to the left arm or jaw and is more common in men than in women. Angina most often comes on with exertion and goes away with rest or a nitroglycerin pill taken under the tongue, though it can come on at rest. People who get these distress signals are the lucky ones. Typically their doctors will order an angiogram, also called cardiac catheterization, a test that inserts dye into the arteries and illuminates them on a video screen, revealing where blockages are and how big they are (see chapter 4). Sometimes an angiogram reveals several blockages of different sizes in two or three arteries, even a plaque that is blocking 99 percent of the passage in an artery. When the blockage is this extreme, it must be treated to prevent total blockage and a heart attack and to relieve the symptoms of angina. Treatment usually means one of two things: clear out the artery with a stent that pushes the plaque to one side or surgically implant another blood vessel to bypass the blockage.

Unlike stents that move blockages out of the way, coronary bypass surgery creates detours around the blockages in arteries. To create these detours, the cardiac surgeon will often use one of the two arteries that runs down the inside of the chest wall in front of the heart, the *left and right internal mammary arteries.* Most often, the left one is used to create a detour around a blockage in the left anterior descending coronary artery. The cardiac surgeon may also use a piece of vein removed from the patient's leg to make a detour. One end is sewn to the aorta and the other to the coronary artery beyond the blockage. Vein grafts often occlude after a time, however. This may happen in as soon as several days or as long as 20 years or more. Because arterial grafts are more likely to remain open, I (Ed) would rather see my patient get a left or right internal mammary artery graft.

Coronary artery bypass surgery is very effective in relieving angina, but it is major surgery and should not be done just for that reason. Most people with angina get along well, or at least get by, on medications alone. Bypass surgery may be recommended if the angina is not relieved by medications, if the blockage is particularly threatening in the left main coronary artery, or if there are multiple severe blockages in the left anterior descending, circumflex, and right coronary arteries. Bypass surgery is usually chosen over stenting if more than one or two plaques would need stenting.

In a person who already has heart failure because of poor left ventricular function, the risk of surgery is higher, so the cardiologist, cardiac surgeon, and the person should all agree that the benefit from the surgery would be greater than the risk. This question is very difficult to answer. There is reason to believe that people whose left ventricle is working so poorly that it is causing them to have heart failure, and who have multiple blockages of 70 percent or more, yet have no symptoms of angina, might benefit from bypass surgery. The reason is that the bypass will improve the function of the left ventricle, increase the heart's pumping ability as evidenced by a higher ejection fraction, and therefore decrease symptoms of heart failure. The surgery should also prolong the person's life, but we do not know if this is true because there have been no studies of survival rates in people with weakly pumping hearts who had bypass surgery.

The idea behind the surgery for this set of people—those who have a poorly functioning left ventricle who are not experiencing angina despite an artery blockage of 70 percent—is the concept of a *hibernating myocardium*. When there is a severe blockage in a coronary artery, the heart tissue beyond the blockage can hibernate, slowing down its need for oxygen by decreasing function to match the decreased blood flow it is getting. If coronary blood flow is restored to normal, this hibernating heart tissue will again contract normally, improving overall heart function and decreasing the symptoms of heart failure. This has happened in animals and in some patients, but we do not know how common it is. This question is being studied in a large trial.

If your cardiologist recommends coronary artery bypass surgery, ask why and what the alternatives are. Consider all your options carefully before agreeing to this surgery. There are situations where it is clearly indicated, and other situations where the evidence of benefit is not as clear. Discuss this with your cardiologist and the cardiac surgeon. Be sure to understand their reasoning. Then get a second surgeon's opinion at a different hospital. Only when you have educated yourself about this surgery and your other options and fully understand the opinions of the doctors you consulted should you decide what you think is right for you.

Bypass surgery has complications, the worst of which are stroke, heart attack, and even death. These complications occur in 2 percent of cases nationally and vary a good bit from one hospital and one surgeon to another. Before agreeing to the surgery, ask what your surgeon's percentage of complications is and discuss these risks. Depression and memory loss are much more common. In fact, 40 to 50 percent of patients having any type of cardiac surgery may suffer transient depression or memory loss. For some, the loss is long term. It often happens that the sicker you are going into the surgery, the greater your risk of complications.

Typically, you should expect to spend 5 to 7 days in the hospital and another 2 to 4 weeks at home recuperating. You will not feel well and energetic for 1 to 2 months after any major cardiac surgery. You will be left with a scar on your chest that runs the length of your breastbone and another on your legs if vein grafts were used to create the bypass.

If your bypass surgery was done for the right reason, you can feel lucky that you were helped in time, and you should soon feel both relief from your discomfort and a new energy.

VALVE SURGERY

While cholesterol deposits are the bane of arteries, calcium deposits and aging are the enemy of heart valves, making them stiff and unable to open or close properly. Most commonly affected is the aortic valve. Valve disease frequently leads to heart failure. To force blood past this partially open valve, the left ventricle has to pump all the harder and may eventually weaken as a result of overuse. If the valve is replaced, the left ventricle doesn't have to work so hard, and the heart is able to bounce back to normal. Replacement of a defective aortic valve often provides complete relief from heart failure.

Sometimes when the aortic valve does not close properly, blood that was ejected out of the heart leaks, or regurgitates, back into the heart. Blood leaking back into the left ventricle can cause a weakening of the heart muscle because the heart is processing the same blood again, an extra workload.

Timing of surgical intervention for a leaky aortic valve is crucial. The heart can compensate for a variable period before the left ventricle becomes weak. However, once the left ventricle weakens, replacing the valve may come too late for the left ventricle to recuperate. If your surgeon suggests replacing a leaking valve, be sure to ask if damage has already occurred to your left ventricle and what chance there is that replacing your valve will actually help you. The problem is that if your leaking valve is not replaced, your heart will continue to be damaged, so your doctor's advice most of the time will be to go ahead and replace the valve in the hope that it might make a difference.

What type of valve to use as a replacement—a human valve, a pig valve, or a mechanical valve—depends on many factors. Be sure to discuss this choice with your surgeon before the operation. Each has risks and benefits. The mechanical valve will likely last forever but requires that you take a blood thinner for the rest of your life to prevent blood clots from forming in the valve. The pig valve does not require a blood thinner but does not last as long. This might be just the choice for an older person not expected to live another decade because of age alone or for a young woman anticipating pregnancy, who does not want to use the blood thinner because of risks to the baby. In such a case, the woman needs to accept that the pig valve will eventually have to be replaced with a mechanical valve when she is no longer in her childbearing years.

The human valve works particularly well if the reason for the valve replacement is *endocarditis,* an infection of the person's own valve. Human replacement valves, like the pig valve, tend to last no more than 8 to 10 years, but they appear to be less prone to infection than a pig valve or mechanical valve when used in patients with endocarditis because there is less chance of getting reinfected.

The mitral valve can also become leaky or open only part way. In the developed world, a leaky mitral valve is much more common than a partially open valve. In those parts of the world where rheumatic fever is still common, a partially open valve, known as *mitral stenosis,* remains a common complication. The mitral valve may be replaced or repaired. Of the two, repair is much to be desired if at all possible. This is very delicate surgery and requires a surgeon with expertise and knowledge. Definitely discuss with your surgeon the option of repair rather than replacement. If your surgeon does not feel qualified to offer repair, ask for a recommendation to a surgeon who is competent in that kind of surgery.

VENTRICULAR RESTORATION

In this operation, the surgeon is trying to restore the normal geometry of the left ventricle. The normal left ventricle is a *proloid ellipse,* which is a fancy term for the shape of a football with one end cut off. After a large untreated myocardial infarction, the geometry of the left ventricle becomes much rounder, like a beach ball. This change in shape is associated with heart failure and decreased survival. *Ventricular restoration* seeks to return the left ventricle to a football, thereby relieving heart failure symptoms and improving survival. The surgeon can do this in several different ways, but it is simplest to remove the dead heart tissue that no longer contracts. This operation is most commonly done when a heart attack involved the anterior (front) wall of the heart. Trials of this sort of surgery compared with medical therapy are ongoing. Preliminary results suggest that this may not be as effective as originally thought. Until results of the studies are known, doctors are not yet certain who benefits from this type of surgery and whether benefit can be predicted prior to the operation. In addition, we do not know if bypass surgery alone or bypass surgery plus ventricular restoration is the better operation. This, too, is an area of active research.

PASSIVE RESTRAINT

If the change in geometry from a football with one end cut off to a beach ball is bad for people with coronary disease, wouldn't preventing this shape change in the first place be of benefit? This is the concept behind various means of *passive restraint.* Think of a meshlike device that can be fitted like a girdle around the left ventricle and you have the right idea. This device is still experimental and has not been approved by the Food and Drug Administration. Only time will tell if this procedure will produce benefits.

Not all surgeons are equally gifted, and not all hospitals have the same results. Some surgeons are truly capable of real magic. Some hospitals simply have much more experience with cardiac surgery and often better results. The surgeon plays an absolutely critical role. The nurses and technicians who care for you after surgery will also make a crucial difference. The experience of the entire team of doctors, nurses, technicians, and others affects how well you will do after surgery.

Some states publish heart surgery statistics by hospital or by both hospital and surgeon. Ask your surgeon, state health department, or Medicare office if statistics are available in your state. Ask why your cardiologist is referring you to this particular surgeon at that specific hospital. It is not only acceptable, but it is very important for you to ask surgeons about their experience and their hospital's statistics. In a true emergency, there simply will not be the time for such research. If time is less of an issue, it pays to look into where you should have the surgery done and who you want to do the surgery.

Surgery can be of great benefit to the right person with heart failure. Coronary artery bypass surgery is commonly performed with low risk and excellent results. The questions of whether it benefits those with heart failure and poor left ventricular function due to coronary disease remain open. Valve surgery is less commonly performed but has excellent outcomes. Both operations would often be preferable to heart transplantation. Ventricular restoration and passive restraint using a meshlike device both remain experimental. Expect that there will be new surgical options for people with heart failure in the years ahead.

9

Device Treatments for the Critically Ill

Sometimes drugs and biventricular pacemakers are not enough to help a very sick heart recover. Then a person may need a device as a means of support until a donor heart becomes available for transplantation. Most common are *ventricular assist devices,* which take over much of the pumping function of the failing heart but do not replace the heart. Less common is the total artificial heart, which, as the name suggests, replaces the heart with a mechanical one.

Mechanical hearts and ventricular assist devices may conjure up the image of the Tin Man, who wanted a heart in the *Wizard of Oz*. But there is no fantasy involved. Every year I (Ed) see people saved by such devices. They are not for everyone, but they can be magical when used in the right person.

Very rarely one of these devices will be used as a bridge to recovery, to the point when the patient's own heart improves enough to no longer need it. Occasionally, a device becomes *destination therapy* until the end of life in a person when there is no plan for heart transplantation, usually because there is a reason transplantation would not work well.

The expertise needed to surgically implant these devices and follow patients afterward is usually found in institutions with a commitment to treating heart failure and providing heart transplantation. Look for heart transplant programs, and you will usually find surgeons and cardiologists knowledgeable in ventricular assist devices and total artificial hearts.

VENTRICULAR ASSIST DEVICES

A ventricular assist device can be used to support the right ventricle or, more commonly, the left ventricle. A *left ventricular assist device* is a pump that removes blood from the left ventricle by suction and pumps it into the aorta. It is used when the person's own left ventricle is too weak. In this situation, the right ventricle will push blood to the lungs to pick up oxygen as it normally does. Blood then flows passively back to the left atrium and to the left ventricle. There the left ventricular assist device

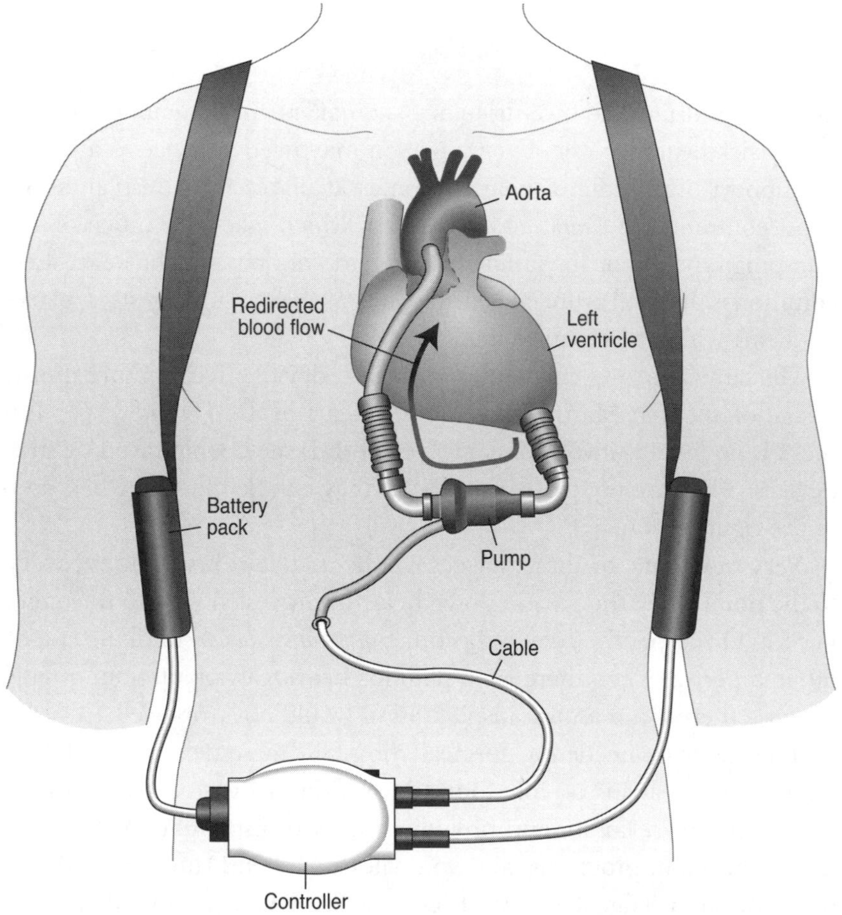

Figure 9.1. Left ventricular assist device. In this device, a rotary pump removes blood from the left ventricle and pumps it into the aorta. This is coordinated via a controller located outside the patient, which can be connected to batteries or to an electrical outlet.

takes over, pumping blood from the left ventricle into the aorta and to the rest of the body. (See figure 9.1.)

Left ventricular assist devices are capable of providing not only normal but greater than normal blood flow if everything works correctly. They can be adjusted to provide the proper blood flow in each patient.

In the rare situation when the right ventricle is too weak, a *right ventricular assist device* may be needed. In this case, the device would take blood from the right ventricle by suction and pump it to the lungs.

Very rarely, a left ventricular assist device and a right ventricular assist device are necessary. This occurs when both the right and left ventricle are too weak. In such cases, a total artificial heart may be a better alternative.

There are many different types of ventricular assist devices. These pumps differ in several ways. The location of the pump may be inside the body or outside the body. It may be driven electrically or pneumatically (by air). The pump may deliver a wave of blood to the body, leading to a pulse with each actuation of the pump, much like the normal heartbeat, or it may deliver continuous blood flow, where there is no pulse and blood is simply moved forward by rotary motion (think of blood being moved by a spinning propeller). These are all differences in the technology of the device. From the perspective of the person with such a device, size, shape, and other issues are probably much more important to their quality of life than the technology involved.

Because the pump on all ventricular assist devices must be controlled, the devices are attached to a controller, which varies in size from a laptop computer to a small bedside table on wheels. The choice of which type of device to use is based on many things, including body size, reason for use, and availability. Since the need to place a device in a patient often happens quickly, the patient and family may not be much involved in any discussion about which device will be used.

Ventricular Assist Devices for Short-Term Support

Ventricular assist devices that are used for short-term support are most often located outside the body, with tubes draining blood from the sick ventricle and injecting blood back into either the aorta (in the case of a left ventricular assist device) or pulmonary artery (in the case of a right ventricular assist device). These pumps are meant for short-term support until the heart recovers and are most often used after cardiac surgery, providing several days or weeks of support. Infection is the major risk, since all these tubes running into the body are potential paths for infectious organisms. All these tubes and machines suddenly surrounding a patient make this a frightening situation for most families.

Ventricular Assist Devices for Long-Term Support

The ventricular assist devices that are used as a bridge to transplantation or as destination therapy most often are much smaller and are contained inside the body, because they may be used for months or years. Most common is a left ventricular assist device. The pump, the size of a grapefruit that is squished to make it more of a disk than a ball, is located under the skin of the abdomen, as are the tubes that drain blood from the left ventricle and pump it into the aorta. The tubes have valves to prevent the backward flow of blood. Only one tube, a *driveline,* exits the skin on the other side of the abdomen from the pump and connects to a power supply and the controller.

People with this type of ventricular assist device may eventually be able to exercise and leave the hospital to await transplantation or, in the case of destination therapy, to learn to live with their new pump. Approximately 70 percent of patients with a left ventricular assist device will survive to transplantation. This is a good outcome when you consider that these people were very sick before the device was inserted.

Continuous Flow Ventricular Assist Devices

The traditional ventricular assist device is big. It is hard to fit a grapefruit-sized pump into the belly of a child or a small adult. For such people, *continuous flow pumps* are available. These pumps are dramatically smaller, about the size and shape of a cigar. They will provide blood flow continuously, rather than as a surge of blood followed by a decrease and then another surge, as the normal heart provides. This results in a lack of a systolic and diastolic blood pressure, because there is no rhythmic surge of blood. The long-term effects of blood flow without a pulse are unknown. The continuous flow ventricular assist devices are newer, so there has been less experience with the use of such pumps. However, they have worked well in my experience. They have become the preferred left ventricular assist device used today (see figure 9.1).

Limitations of Ventricular Assist Devices

The major limitations of the ventricular assist devices are that the driveline must exit the body and be connected to a power source and controller. Batteries allow the user to be away from a fixed power source for up to several hours depending on battery life, but long enough to shower or take a walk outside. In addition, some ventricular assist devices are noisy. There is no hiding from the rest of the world that you have a ventricular assist device. Also, the driveline, and anything else that is external before diving into the body, is a track for infection. Infections in a ventricular assist device are difficult if not impossible to cure but can often be contained with antibiotics. They may prove to be fatal.

Some ventricular assist devices are prone to develop blood clots inside the pump itself or inside the tubes that lead to and from the pump. In the case of a left ventricular assist device, clots that break off will lodge in the brain, causing a stroke, or elsewhere in the body, causing sudden lack of blood flow wherever the clot lodges. Because of this risk, with some ventricular assist devices, the person must receive anticoagulants to decrease the stickiness of the blood and thereby help prevent formation of blood clots. Finally, like any humanmade machine, these devices can break, with often catastrophic results. Some ventricular assist devices are more durable than others, and some are less prone to forming blood clots.

There is one good trial of left ventricular assist devices in people who were very sick but not candidates for heart transplantation. They were not candidates mostly because they were too old or had kidney disease likely to limit life expectancy after transplantation. In this multicenter trial, 129 people were randomized to receive either a left ventricular assist device (68 people) or continued medical therapy (61 people). The one-year survival of the people who got a left ventricular assist device was 48 percent, while the survival of those on medications alone was 26 percent. At two years, the survival was 26 percent and 8 percent respectively. Clearly we are not talking about a device likely to keep someone alive for five years. But it will add months of extra life in most cases. In addition, quality of life was improved in those who had a left ventricular assist device. More recent improvements to the devices have likely improved the survival rate, but they still do not rival heart transplantation.

Why would someone consider using a ventricular assist device? In my experience, these people are incredibly ill, often far too ill to read this chapter. The device is the only means to bridge them either to a heart transplant or, rarely, recovery. Most people who get a ventricular assist device, therefore, will end up with a heart transplant. I do not think that destination therapy is, in general, a good idea. Survival is short and quality of life is better, but not dramatically better than living with heart failure, largely because the person is so dependent on the technology. Pictures of people fly fishing with a left ventricular assist device capture the reality for only a few. The rest will lead much more limited lifestyles.

Timing of device placement is important. Survival is not good if the person is too sick before the operation, and yet the person needs to be sick enough to need one. This is often a tricky decision, just as the surgery to implant the device itself is very risky.

TOTAL ARTIFICIAL HEART

The *total artificial heart,* which has been the source of intense research for almost four decades, has several advantages over the ventricular assist device. Most recently approved by the Food and Drug Administration in September 2006, it is completely implantable and is charged through the skin without the use of a driveline. This is a significant milestone in the development of all such devices and will decrease infection risk as well as make life easier for the person who gets the heart. The device is approved for destination therapy. The company has not yet applied for approval to market it as a bridge to transplantation, but surgeons use it also for this reason.

The other models of artificial hearts are both big, in fact too big to fit inside many people. The next generation will be smaller. One of the large models is approved for use as a bridge to transplantation and the other as destination therapy. Another advantage to the total artificial heart is that it will replace the heart entirely, so those whose hearts are weak on both sides will not need two pumps, one to support the right and another to support the left.

It will be interesting to watch what happens with the use of the total artificial heart compared to ventricular assist devices. To date, many more ventricular assist devices have been placed because they were simply more durable and the technology was better. This may reverse in the future.

LIVING WITH A POWER-DRIVEN HEART

Both a ventricular assist device and a total artificial heart are designed to allow you to recuperate, get stronger, and live better until a donor heart becomes available. Rarely, they are used to prolong life in people who won't receive heart transplantation. Whether or not you are awaiting a transplant, you will benefit from exercise rehabilitation to improve muscle strength and conditioning. You should try to eat a healthy diet, although sometimes the grapefruit-sized pump will limit the ability of your stomach to expand and accept large meals. Eating multiple small meals may be the answer.

You will need very close follow-up by the team that placed the device. The follow-up requires a level of technology and expertise located in only a few places. If you live far from one of these centers, you may need to move closer.

Most of my patients, but not all by any means, who had a ventricular assist device tell me they would do it again. Ventricular assist devices and total artificial hearts can be magical, almost like raising Lazarus from the dead. They represent in many ways the pinnacle of technology used to prolong survival and improve quality of life. But they have a price. Such therapy is expensive not only in dollars but also in the energy and emotional commitment demanded of the person who has one, the person's family, and the medical care system as well.

10

Getting a New Heart

Getting a new heart is the epitome of getting a second chance. It is awesome. People plagued by shortness of breath who barely had the energy to get out of bed can, with a new heart, go back to work, drive a car, play tennis, take care of children or grandchildren, garden, and run errands unaccompanied. A heart transplant recipient can go from slowly dying to fully living.

Because it is a high-risk surgery that is difficult for everyone involved, however, a heart transplant is the treatment of last resort. If you surrender your biological heart for a new heart from a donor, it is because no other treatments are working, and your own heart has failed so badly that it is causing severe distress and will only get worse.

Mary Pitz, who lives on a Pennsylvania farm, was 65 when her cardiologist referred her for a heart transplant in 2000. She had idiopathic cardiomyopathy, and the pacemaker she had worn for 8 years was no longer helping. She describes how she felt: "Very, very tired, no energy whatsoever, very short of breath." Her cardiologist said she had 2 to 5 years to live and asked if she wanted to have a heart transplant.

For Mrs. Pitz, the decision was simple: "On the one hand you have death; on the other you have a longer life." She chose the chance for a longer life, explaining, "I've always felt positive about this." Today she is still the kind of woman who stands out, with beautiful short white hair framing soft facial features. Her donor, age 19, died in a Labor Day traffic accident, and Mrs. Pitz was transplanted the next day.

Seven years after getting her new heart, she talked about the energy she has and how she enjoys spinning and weaving, going to craft guild meetings, and getting together with a gardening group. She has no trouble crouching to pull up weeds, enjoys cooking, and makes a point of spending individual time with her eight grandchildren, going on long shopping and lunch outings with each one. She and her husband went to Alaska for two weeks in the summer of 2007, and they frequently exchange life on their 32-acre farm for a visit to the mountains, where they keep a trailer. What an incredible turnaround in her life from those days before she got a new heart and had no energy. "They want you to live your life," Mrs. Pitz said of her heart transplant team.

During my 10 years as director of the Johns Hopkins Heart Transplant Service, I (Ed) walked with over 200 people as they went through the process of being evaluated for and eventually receiving a heart transplant. Their stories are every bit as compelling as Mary Pitz's story. Nothing has been more fulfilling for me as a physician than caring for these patients. I get to feel the highs of their successes and the lows of their disappointments. Through it all, I sense how lucky they truly are to have been given a second chance.

THE PROGRESS OF HEART TRANSPLANTATION

The first human heart transplant on December 3, 1967, shocked the world of medicine and the public. In those early years of transplantation, insurmountable problems of overwhelming infection and rejection of the new heart as foreign tissue prevented heart recipients from living very long. Stanford University led research in preventing rejection and developing immunotherapy that transformed heart transplantation from an experiment to standard treatment for late-stage heart disease. While rejection and infection are still problems to watch for and treat, doctors and patients today are very grateful to those pioneering doctors and patients who brought us to this point of high expectation for living well with a new heart. Today about 3,300 patients are on a waiting list for a heart transplant. The majority of recipients are between the ages of 50 and 64, although heart surgeons have placed new hearts in babies and in patients in their seventies.

Getting a new heart is an extraordinary gift, a privilege, and a daily responsibility. The person who says yes to a heart transplant also says yes to a lifetime of medical procedures and daily medications. Not every transplant is successful. There are serious risks involved during and after

Table 10.1. Heart Transplantation Survival Rates

	Percentage of transplant recipients who survived	
Number of years	*Males*	*Females*
1	85	85
3	78.9	76.1
5	72	68.5

Source: Scientific Registry of Transplant Recipients, UStransplant.org

the surgery, and 10 percent of recipients die within three months of receiving the new heart. The one-year survival rate is 85 percent (see table 10.1). Ten years after transplant, 51 percent of heart recipients are alive. If this 10-year figure doesn't seem impressive, remember that heart transplants are offered to the sickest heart failure patients who, without getting a new heart, might have a 50 percent one-year survival rate.

To find out more about survival rates following transplantation at the various transplant centers in the United States, go to www.ustransplant.org. Be careful not to add an "s" to that Web site address. A commercial Web site appears when you key in the plural form of ustransplant. The correct Web site will say "Scientific Registry of Transplant Recipients" at the top of the page.

WHO NEEDS A HEART TRANSPLANT?

People who are put on a waiting list for a heart transplant often are unable to do even the simplest of physical tasks, like bathing, without encountering difficulty breathing. They may even be short of breath while resting, and often they are so ill that they are confined to bed or hospitalized. Their heart problems may be severe coronary artery disease that cannot be treated with coronary bypass surgery, severe valvular heart disease, or congenital heart problems that are causing major symptoms or life-threatening arrhythmias that cannot be controlled. Sometimes, technical problems make other surgery not an option. Sometimes, medications just don't work. A heart transplant is only for those very sick patients who are not helped by other treatments.

WHO GETS A NEW HEART?

Given the limited number of donor hearts, not all people who need a heart transplant will receive one. About 2,300 of the 3,300 on a waiting list will get a new heart, but 600 others on the list will die before a donor heart becomes available. Some stay waiting. Some get better and are removed from the list because they no longer need a new heart. Some are removed from the list because they develop another problem, such as cancer, and are no longer candidates. Ethically, this is an issue of utilizing a scarce resource, donor hearts, so heart transplantation is offered to the neediest and those most likely to do well.

In deciding who gets a new heart, the first question to be answered is this: Does the person really need a heart transplant? Doctors first look to see if anything else can be done to improve the person's condition short of heart transplantation. Being very sick is not *by itself* a reason to get a heart transplant. Many people who come in to their first cardiologist's visit or hospital stay with severe symptoms are scared and worried that their heart is about to give out and that they may die. And if they weren't worried before, when I tell them they have heart failure, they often think that means they will die unless they get a new heart. But many very sick people have found that, once they are on the right medications or device therapies, they can resume their regular active lives. Five million people in the United States are living with heart failure. Of these, heart transplantation is the answer for much less than 1 percent.

Once it is determined that a patient cannot be helped by drug or device treatments, doctors try to answer the second big question: Will this patient do well with a heart transplant? Each potential recipient undergoes a heart transplant evaluation at a center that performs the operation. The evaluation includes screening for other life-threatening problems, ensuring that other factors aren't likely to limit life expectancy beyond the heart condition. Examples are cancer or failure of another organ like the liver or kidneys. Continued tobacco use, illicit drug use, and alcohol abuse also predict poor outcomes following transplantation. Potential recipients are told to stop these uses before the evaluation begins.

These days most programs will consider healthy 70-year-olds. The age of the recipient and other factors that decide who is considered a good risk for a new heart are left up to the individual centers. When I first became involved in heart transplantation, the cut-off age was 55 years.

There are at least two important nonmedical factors considered as part of estimating how well a prospective transplant patient will do:

1. Does the patient have a strong support system? At Johns Hopkins, we often tell potential recipients that we "transplant families, not people." The medical regimen after heart transplantation is complex, and the heart recipient needs support to get to all the appropriate appointments and take all the correct medications. This support often comes from family members but could come from close personal friends willing to serve in this role.
2. Will the patient be willing to follow a daily regimen of 10 to 15 medications without which he or she would develop serious problems, even die? Potential recipients who have a track record of not following medical advice are not considered appropriate candidates for a transplant.

Although the evaluation varies from one transplant center to another, you should expect to be seen by a cardiologist, a cardiac surgeon, a social worker, and a transplant coordinator. You will have a lot of blood drawn from your arm for testing, and a right heart catheterization will be done to measure pressures in the heart and lungs. In this 30-minute procedure, performed in the hospital under local anesthesia, a tube smaller than a straw is inserted into the heart, usually through the right internal jugular vein, located in the neck. This is done to measure pressure in the lungs.

The lung pressure we measure is elevated in people with severe heart failure in need of heart transplantation. In general, the normal right ventricle of a donor heart is not able to respond to the high pressures in the lungs of someone with severe heart failure. If faced with such high pressures, the new right ventricle may fail to pump adequate blood to the lungs simply because it cannot generate the needed pressure to push blood through them. Usually, elevated lung pressure will normalize rapidly with a new heart. Sometimes, however, the elevated lung pressure leads to potentially permanent changes or scarring in the lungs that will take weeks to reverse. Because of this, the pressure does not fall immediately, and the right ventricle cannot handle the elevated pressure. This can be life threatening, and although we have medications to lower the elevated lung pressure, they sometimes do not work as well as we would like.

If the pressure in the lungs is too high, the person may be given a medication to see if normal or near normal lung pressure can be achieved. The effect of the medication lasts only about 30 minutes, but if the pressure falls, that shows us that the pressure would very likely also fall once the patient gets a new heart, and the new donor heart would be able to handle the increased pressures in the lungs because this would be a temporary situation. If the medication does not cause the pressure to fall and we believe that the lung scarring will not reverse, we consider a heart-lung transplant. Or we may place a left ventricular assist device to see if long-term improvement in left ventricular function and relief from heart failure will lower the lung pressure and reverse the lung scarring. Given time, the right ventricle can often adjust to the elevated pressure, and sometimes the pressure will fall slowly in some recipients.

After the preliminary screening is completed, the transplant team will meet to discuss your case and decide whether to offer you the opportunity to go on the waiting list for a new heart.

I've been telling you what to expect from the heart transplantation team that will evaluate you, but you are a partner in this decision. If you are offered the opportunity to go on a heart transplant waiting list, you will, of course, want to weigh the risk and the expectation of receiving a new heart and a new life against the risk and expectation of keeping your diseased heart. Before agreeing to a heart transplant, satisfy yourself that you have no other option that can significantly improve and extend your life. Ask questions. Be sure you understand your options.

As part of making such a supremely important decision, you would be wise to get the opinion of at least one other board-certified cardiologist who specializes in heart failure. If you are well enough, you may want to get the second opinion from a doctor who works in a different medical center, who is not a close colleague of your doctor, and who trained in a different hospital. In other words, you're looking for independent judgment from well-qualified, seasoned experts. Ask each doctor to review your medical history, examine you, and give a recommendation for your best treatment. Some people have more time and resources to consider this decision than others. If you are very sick and have found a nationally recognized transplant center that performs many transplants every year, that may be enough for you.

When you meet with members of the team at the center where you may get your new heart, ask questions about the surgery and what to expect immediately after and for the long term. You may want to ask if you can talk with a couple of people who have already had heart transplants, to learn how their lives are different with new hearts. Discuss your options with family, close friends, and your doctor. Then, if your medical team decides you are a candidate for a heart transplant, the decision is yours to make.

Before your name goes on the waiting list, more testing will be done to answer these questions.

- Blood type: A donor heart has to match the recipient's blood type.
- Past infections, including cytomegalovirus infection (CMV) and the presence of HIV. People with HIV will not get a new heart because they have a higher risk of dying after the transplant than do recipients who do not have HIV. This may change as the prognosis of those with HIV is improving. Screening for CMV infection is done to tell the medical team who will need a drug to prevent this infection after the transplant.

THE NEW HEART

If the transplant team decides you need a heart transplant and are a good candidate for the operation, and you decide to proceed, your name will be placed on the regional heart transplant waiting list. The median wait for a heart transplant for the years 2001–2006 was 5.6 months. While each transplant center keeps its own waiting list, the one that really counts is the one maintained by the United Network for Organ Sharing, or UNOS (see www.unos.org). Each of over 100 areas of the country is served by an independent organ procurement organization, or OPO. Hospitals call the OPO when a brain-dead patient who is a potential heart donor is identified.

In a heart transplant, a person's diseased heart is replaced with the heart of a donor who has suffered brain death. In brain death, usually caused by a severe trauma such as a car accident or a large stroke, the brain has no function at all, and this inability to function is permanent. Medical tests can prove the brain has ceased to function. Yet the brain-dead person's heart and lungs can continue functioning with the help of a machine that breathes for the person. During this window of time, which is usually a matter of days, the person's heart stays alive and healthy.

Donation of a heart must be made freely and without coercion. The wish to donate is usually indicated by a prior written agreement from the person, such as with a signed organ donor card, or else the immediate family grants permission.

The local OPO will send a representative to examine the potential donor and make sure the donor heart and other organs are acceptable for transplantation. The donor cannot have a disease such as HIV or leukemia that could be spread to the heart recipient, and the heart will be examined by echocardiography to see that it works well. Donor hearts typically come from younger people, although hearts have come from people who are in their seventies.

If the heart passes inspection as a donor heart, the local OPO contacts UNOS, and an algorithm identifies the potential recipient within a certain geographical area. The algorithm is based on blood type, body size, severity of illness, and time on the waiting list. Body size is used to make sure the heart is not too large or too small. The sickest patients and those who have waited the longest are given priority. The OPO then contacts the transplant center that listed the potential recipient, and a physician from that center calls the recipient. If the person is unable to be transplanted immediately, the algorithm is run again, and a new name is generated. This new person may be at the same transplant center or another transplant center in the region. In any case, the goal is to make the selection in a fair and equitable manner.

The race is then on. The donor heart will be usable for only a short time. Once removed from the donor, the donor heart must be used within about four hours or it will not function well. So things move quickly. Transplantation may occur at any time, including in the middle of the night, when operating rooms are immediately available. The donor is brought to the operating room of the hospital where he died, and the organs to be donated are surgically removed. A surgeon comes from each hospital where a transplant will take place to remove the organ that will be transplanted. The heart is placed in a liquid solution in a plastic bag, and the bag is put on ice and moved quickly to another operating room, perhaps in a different city or even a different state, where the recipient is ready for his new heart. Dr. John V. Conte, director of heart and heart-lung transplantation at Hopkins, says that while the new heart is en route, the patient who will receive the new heart is prepared, but the surgeon waits until the donor heart arrives in the operating room before starting to remove the patient's biological heart. The surgeon has to know that the new heart is at hand before starting to remove the patient's heart, because the courier bringing the new heart could be involved in an accident or a long traffic delay or somehow not get the heart to the surgeon at the expected time. So all is ready and waiting when the doors open and the new heart arrives.

Then the heart transplant begins.

The Surgery

Preparation for heart transplant surgery is necessarily rushed. The surgeon, a nurse, and the anesthesiologist will talk to you. Some blood will be drawn, and a chest x-ray and electrocardiogram done. The surgery lasts between 4 and 12 hours. As soon as the general anesthesia takes effect, a tube is placed down your throat into your windpipe. The other end of the tube is attached to a ventilator, which will breathe for you; this is necessary because the anesthetic includes high doses of narcotics to prevent you from feeling pain during the surgery as well as a muscle-paralyzing agent to keep your body still—a big help to the surgeon. The paralyzing agent stops you from breathing on your own, and that is why you are connected to the ventilator. After the surgeon opens your chest and exposes your heart, the ventilator is turned off. Now a heart-lung bypass machine is connected to you. It will both breathe for you and circulate blood throughout your body, avoiding your heart and taking its place, while your biological heart is removed and your new heart is put in place. The surgeon connects your new heart to the aorta, pulmonary artery, and superior and inferior vena cava. (See figure 10.1.)

The principal risks of heart transplant surgery are the same as for any heart surgery: stroke, heart attack, and death. These complications occur in about 5 percent of the surgeries. The major risk unique to heart transplantation is that sometimes, for a wide variety of reasons, the new heart fails to work properly. This rare (less than 2 percent of heart transplants) and catastrophic situation often results in death.

If all goes well, you will be awake and removed from the breathing machine within a day or so. You might spend three or four days in the intensive care unit, and then go home in about a week.

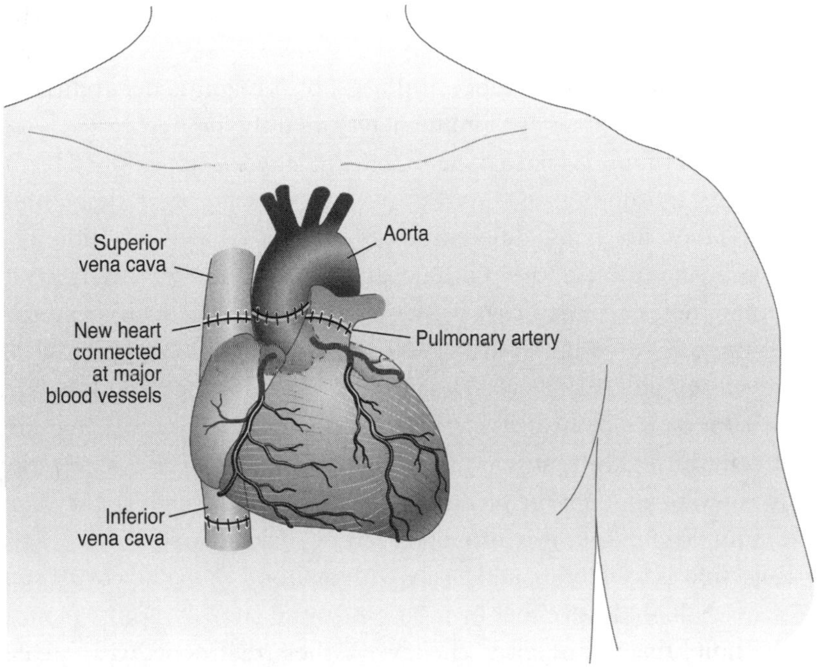

Figure 10.1. Heart transplantation. The new heart is connected by sutures to the superior vena cava, inferior vena cava, pulmonary artery, aorta, and a rim of left atrial tissue including the pulmonary veins (not depicted).

Within a week or so after receiving their new heart, the vast majority of heart recipients feel better and are able to do more than they did before surgery. However, they will be taking just as many medications as they did before surgery, and they will remain tied very closely to the medical system for follow-up care. Getting a new organ, especially a heart, is very different from other surgeries. After many surgeries, such as the removal of a diseased appendix or a noncancerous tumor, the health problem is solved, and the person quickly moves on. For heart transplant patients, when the operation ends, new problems are just beginning.

From this point onward, the primary problem is often a balancing act between rejection and infection. Both are most common in the first six months. After the first year, both are uncommon but not rare. As your body gets used to your new heart, your doctors will be able to decrease the dose of the immunosuppressant medications you must take.

Managing Rejection

Rejection is the body's attempt to rid itself of foreign tissue, in this case the new heart. The body will immediately identify the new heart as foreign and will mount a fatal attack on it if the attack is not stopped by the use of immunosuppressants—powerful drugs that suppress the immune system. There are many different drugs used to prevent rejection, and other drugs are used to treat it if it occurs. To prevent rejection, typically a combination of three drugs is used, a corticosteroid such as prednisone, and two other immunosuppressants. These three drugs have different actions and side effects. Despite this immunosuppressant therapy, 40 percent of recipients will have an episode of rejection that requires treatment during the first year after the transplant. The risk of rejection is increased in younger recipients and in females, especially if they have had multiple children. It is also increased in African Americans.

Rejection is usually treated easily with a short course of corticosteroids at very high doses either by mouth or intravenously. Eighty percent of the time, this treatment is effective. Other treatments with greater side effects include antibodies directed against certain white blood cells required for rejection. Most rejection is successfully treated and leaves no lasting effects on the heart.

The medications used to prevent and treat rejection cause multiple side effects. The side effects of corticosteroids such as prednisone include diabetes mellitus, osteoporosis, obesity, acne, stomach ulcers, high blood pressure, and depression. Corticosteroid use also leads to a characteristic change in appearance. The face becomes rounder, and a hump of tissue develops where the neck meets the back. Other immunosuppressants also cause characteristic side effects. Cyclosporine and tacrolimus may cause kidney problems, high blood pressure, liver problems, swollen gums, increased hair growth in areas other than the top of the head, high cholesterol, and elevated potassium levels. Mycophenolate mofetil may cause nausea, vomiting, diarrhea, loss of appetite, stomach ulcers, abdominal pain, and a decrease in the white blood cell count. These side effects are manageable, and most people do fine. Close contact with the transplant center is required to manage side effects; the dose of the medication may need to be adjusted, or a drug may need to be discontinued and another drug taken in its place.

Doctors try to keep a step ahead of rejection by looking for it when it is easier to treat, before it causes symptoms. To check for rejection, a cardiologist will take a biopsy of the new heart. A heart biopsy, done as an outpatient procedure that takes about 30 minutes, is less scary than it sounds. Using local anesthetic to numb the area of the neck that is entered, a cardiologist will snake a surgical instrument called a bioptome down the right jugular vein of the neck and, under x-ray or echocardiographic guidance, pass it down into the right ventricle of the heart. A tiny piece of heart muscle about the size of a grain of rice is removed from the right ventricle. Several samples are taken for a pathologist to examine under a microscope.

A heart biopsy is a mildly painful procedure, especially getting the local numbing medicine in place. For many recipients, it is like going to the dentist to get a cavity filled. The difference is that it will be done frequently—as often as every week or two for the first month or so. If no rejection is found, the frequency is decreased with time. After about the first year, some transplant centers perform these biopsies only if they suspect that a patient might be beginning to have rejection. Other centers continue to do "surveillance biopsies" for many years. It is not unusual for a patient to have thirty or more heart biopsies over the years.

Managing Infection

The corollary to all this immunosuppression is infection. If the immune system is suppressed, infection will sometimes follow. While undergoing heavy immunosuppression, such as within the first six months of surgery or after treatment of rejection, heart transplant recipients are prone to infection with unusual organisms. Infection may be viral, bacterial, fungal, or even parasitic. A person with a new heart will take prophylactic antibiotics or antiviral drugs to prevent infection from some of these organisms.

In addition to infection with unusual organisms, heart transplant recipients are more susceptible to all the usual infections that can affect anyone in the population. Most recipients will be treated for infection at some time after their heart transplant. Nearly 40 percent will require hospitalization for an infection, and most will do just fine with therapy. However, for about 6 percent of heart transplant recipients, infection does not respond to antibiotics. Sometimes the organism is resistant to the antibiotics, and sometimes the infection is overwhelming. The result is that the patient dies. Most of the time we don't know why.

An example of a serious infectious threat is CMV, a common virus that many of us have been infected with. In transplant recipients, it can be a major problem if it infects the gut, lungs, brain, liver, or bloodstream. Early diagnosis and treatment are critical. For this reason, heart transplant recipients must take fever seriously. *Contact your transplant center immediately if you develop a fever.* A typical definition of fever is a temperature greater than 100.2 degrees Fahrenheit.

Other Common Problems

Within 5 years of the transplant, 34 percent of recipients will develop diabetes mellitus, 33 percent kidney problems, 94 percent hypertension, and 86 percent high cholesterol. These are partly to be expected as side effects from the medications, especially kidney problems and diabetes mellitus. High blood pressure and high cholesterol are common before heart transplant and are made worse after transplantation by the medications used to prevent rejection. Skin cancer is also common and likely a side effect of prior sun exposure plus immunosuppression. Keep in close contact with the transplant center, whose staff can help you with prompt recognition of problems and appropriate treatment.

The most feared complication of cardiac transplantation is the development of accelerated atherosclerosis in the transplanted heart. This occurs in about 30 percent of patients within 5 years of the transplant. This is not the typical form of atherosclerosis, and it doesn't look the same under a microscope, having far less cholesterol and fat accumulation than the standard form. It occurs much more rapidly and can involve the entire length of the coronary arteries, unlike typical atherosclerosis, which develops over a lifetime and tends to occur in patches. (Recall that coronary arteries are transplanted along with the donor heart.) Accelerated atherosclerosis develops only in the transplanted heart and related arteries; it does not occur throughout the recipient's body.

The cause of accelerated atherosclerosis is unclear, but a common reaction to disruption or injury of the innermost lining of the coronary arteries—the endothelial cells—appears to play the most important role. Injury to endothelial cells most likely occurs when the donor heart is removed. Treatment is difficult. Sometimes angioplasty and stenting can be performed. Other times, coronary bypass might be recommended.

If the coronary arteries are involved from beginning to end, these options are not viable and sometimes repeat transplantation is considered. Medical therapy alone is not as good as we would like. Prevention is also difficult, although some believe that standard cholesterol-lowering drugs such as statins may help. Accelerated atherosclerosis is the major stumbling block to long-term survival and is an area of active research.

IN THE LONG TERM

How Can You Expect to Feel?

Once you get beyond the immediate post-transplant phase, if all goes well, you will feel better, likely much better. Mrs. Pitz says that, for her, a benchmark was when the staples were removed. This is usually done about 7 to 10 days after the surgery. Another big benchmark came in two months. "I could drive eight weeks after the transplant," she remembers. "When you can get out and move about, it makes a big difference." Ninety percent of patients will have no activity limitations. You will do more, have fewer symptoms, and enjoy life more. "There's a settling-in period," she explains. "It takes about two years until you feel really on top of things."

Recipients can return to work and exercise—a few have even played professional sports. Travel is usually not a problem. A return to normal or near normal sexual function is not unusual. Women have carried and delivered children following transplantation, and these children appear unaffected by the medical regimen required of their mother.

How Can You Help Yourself?

Make sure you understand directions, and follow them carefully. Keep a list of your medications with you at all times, and take them faithfully. Get routine follow-up and participate in a support group for transplant recipients. These steps will help you in the long run.

Organization is key. Keep a daily written record of your blood pressure, pulse, blood sugar (if diabetic), and weight for at least the first six months after the transplant. Show your recorded health stats to the doctors and nurses caring for you at each visit to the heart transplant center after your operation.

Do everything within your control to keep this new heart working as well as possible. Report fevers, which might be a sign of infection, to your heart transplant team. Eat a healthy diet (see chapter 12), exercise regularly (see chapter 13), avoid tobacco, and consume no more than a glass or two of alcohol a day. Do not drink grapefruit juice, which slows the elimination of both cyclosporine and tacrolimus.

Many fellow heart recipients share your goal of a better, longer life and your sense of awe at getting this second chance. There are 20,000 people in the United States alone living with transplanted hearts today.

"I feel so good most of the time that I don't have to consciously think about it," says Mary Pitz. And yet, she says, a new heart is a gift you never forget. She has always felt that her heart is Hispanic, information she thinks the heart conveyed to her. "I always think of myself as 'we,'" Mrs. Pitz says with a warm smile. "I take the age of my heart and my age and add them together and divide by two and that's how old I am. My age is 48."

11

Future Therapies

For the past 30 years or more, the pace of research into cardiovascular illness not only has been rapid, it has also changed how we diagnose and treat heart disease. I (Ed) expect this rapid pace to continue, as long as our government continues to fund medical research. Predicting where this research will take us is nearly impossible, and unexpected discoveries and advances are part of the excitement.

MAKING THE DIAGNOSIS: CT ANGIOGRAPHY

Today, no single test proves that heart failure is present. Instead, doctors rely on their clinical experience to recognize the signs and symptoms of heart failure. But new methods for diagnosing cardiovascular illness will be developed in the future. And most heart failure patients are asked to undergo diagnostic tests to determine whether coronary disease or something else is causing the heart failure. Diagnostic testing for them and others with heart disease is about to get easier and quicker.

Medical science is right on the cusp of supplanting three standard heart tests with one that will give as much or more detailed information than those three combined. The new test is a 320-slice *computerized tomographic* (CT) scan that will provide images of the heart and arteries in only a second or two. When perfected, for most heart patients this test will replace echocardiography, cardiac catheterization, and nuclear perfusion imaging—a test that shows how coronary artery blockages are affecting the heart.

In the new CT scan, contrast material is injected into a vein in the patient's arm and travels to the heart. The patient is then rolled into a doughnutlike machine where x-rays are used to take pictures of the heart and coronary arteries. The x-ray signals feed into a computer. The currently available 64-slice CT angiographic scans (see chapter 4) provide excellent views of the structure and function of the heart, much like echocardiography, as well as fine details of the coronary arteries. The 320-slice CT scanner, a very expensive machine available now at only a few institutions, adds even greater detail of the coronary arteries as well as an assessment of how significant a partial coronary blockage is at rest and with stress.

This information is currently obtained with a combination of both cardiac catheterization and nuclear perfusion imaging. During a nuclear perfusion test, a small amount of radioactive material, such as thallium or more commonly sestamibi, is injected into a vein during a stress test. These substances move through the blood and are taken up by that portion of the heart that has good blood flow. If one or more of the coronary arteries are blocked, the portion of the heart supplied by that coronary artery does not take up the substance as well. The cardiac catheterization gives information about the anatomy, and the nuclear perfusion scan provides information about the significance of the blockages seen at cardiac catheterization. The new 320-slice CT angiography can provide similar information in a single study.

The problem with the current versions of the 320-slice CT scanners is that they provide so much information, it is difficult to deal with all of it without a small army of computer technicians to manipulate the data so that physicians can view and understand what the scan says about a patient's heart. When widely available, however, this scan will be quickly done and nearly painless. Consumers need to bear in mind, however, that this newest CT scanner for hearts is a very expensive machine, and that a hospital or group of doctors that owns one will likely want to make frequent use of it to pay for its cost. Not all cardiologists agree on its usefulness. As with all tests you get, be sure to understand why you are getting the test and what your doctor hopes to learn from it, and make sure you agree that the test is worth taking. Not all heart patients need all three tests that this one test would replace.

TREATMENT: NEW DRUGS

In terms of medical therapy, there will be new medications and new uses for old medications. While currently available drugs for heart failure do a good job already, cardiologists are eagerly awaiting some promising medications that will be as effective or more so, but with fewer or even no side effects.

Diuretics and Diureticlike Drugs

More effective diuretics will remove fluid without altering kidney function or lowering sodium, potassium, and magnesium concentrations in the blood. *Arginine vasopressin* is a hormone released by the brain's pituitary gland in a person who has heart failure. It causes fluid retention and a low serum sodium concentration. While we emphasize in this book that you should avoid high amounts of sodium in your diet, arginine vasopressin changes the *concentration* of sodium in your blood. The two factors—consumption and concentration—may not be directly related. If you put a teaspoon of salt into an 8-ounce glass of water, you can measure the concentration of sodium in that water. If you now add another 8 ounces of water without adding more salt, you will decrease the concentration of sodium. This happens in heart failure. Some people with particularly severe heart failure and under the influence of arginine vasopressin retain fluid to a greater extent than they retain sodium. With that, the sodium concentration in the blood falls. This indicates extensive fluid retention.

In people with heart failure, low sodium is associated with a higher hospital readmission rate and a higher mortality rate. Several drugs being studied block the arginine vasopressin receptor, causing water but not sodium to leave the body. Tolvaptan is one of these drugs. In a 2004 trial in which either tolvaptan or a placebo was randomly given in addition to the standard therapy to 319 patients admitted with heart failure, tolvaptan improved many of the signs and symptoms of heart failure without causing any adverse effects. There was no effect on long-term mortality or rehospitalization for heart failure, however. An FDA advisory panel recommended approval for tolvaptan in June 2008 for the treatment of *hyponatremia* (low sodium).

Natriuretic Peptides

Brain natriuretic peptide (BNP) is more than a biomarker in heart failure. It is also used to relieve fluid retention and improve heart pressures in people with heart failure. Many other natriuretic peptides do the same things, but human BNP is the best studied and is available currently to treat people admitted to the hospital with *acute decompensated* heart failure. People in this condition have symptoms of heart failure, such as shortness of breath and edema, which are much worse than their usual baseline symptoms and severe enough to warrant admission to the hospital for treatment. BNP helps relieve their congestion and improve other symptoms. However, there have been concerns that BNP may worsen kidney function and lead to death within 30 days. These findings are controversial and have been the stimulus for further investigation into the clinical use and safety of BNP. Other natriuretic peptides, such as carperitide and urodilantin, are also under investigation and may be either more potent or have fewer side effects than BNP, or both.

Drugs that Protect Kidney Function

Adenosine is a building block of DNA that increases the diameter of blood vessels, thereby lowering the pressure within them. Pressure is the force of the blood against the walls of the vessel. Adenosine receptor antagonists are drugs that block receptors for adenosine and may increase urine production without creating the decline in kidney function caused by other diuretics. While adenosine receptors are located widely throughout the body, they are found especially in the kidneys and in the vessels that go to the kidneys, where they influence kidney blood flow and urine production. Blockers of the adenosine receptors located in the kidney not only increase urine production without harming kidney function, they also don't interfere with potassium excretion. Most of these drugs are so new that they do not yet have names and are only referred to by numbers, such as KW-3902.

Drugs that Affect Hormonal Balance

Drugs that affect thyroid hormone, growth hormone, and a hormone named *erythropoietin* that is secreted by the kidneys are also being studied in people with heart failure. Of these, erythropoietin is generating a lot of interest. It stimulates the production of red blood cells and is used as a treatment for anemia in people with renal failure. Many people with heart failure have anemia as well, and the prevalence of anemia increases with the severity of heart failure. Treating these patients with erythropoietin increases the number of red blood cells as expected and decreases the symptoms of heart failure. Studies are under way to evaluate the effects of erythropoietin therapy on mortality in patients with heart failure.

Just the Beginning

These drugs are just a sample of the many drugs being investigated to improve the lives of people with heart failure. Developing a new drug is a lengthy and expensive process. Much more needs to be done to explore the newer drugs in concert with established therapy for heart failure. In addition, safety—in a real-world population of patients with heart failure and not just in a clinical trial—needs to be examined closely.

TREATMENT: NEW DEVICES

Fluid Removal

In the future greater use will be made of mechanical means to remove excess fluid in heart failure. Doctors will use a simple device that removes fluid quickly, thus relieving symptoms without the detrimental effects that diuretics have on kidney function. The drawback is that all such devices require the placement of intravenous lines, which allow blood to be removed from the patient, the serum strained off, and the blood cells returned to the patient. This *ultrafiltration* takes as long as several hours depending on how much fluid needs to be removed; the intravenous lines are removed after every session, thus decreasing the risk of infection.

Pacemakers and Defibrillators

Better, smaller, and longer lasting pacemakers and implantable cardioverter defibrillators (ICDs) will be developed with more features as manufacturers try to compete for business. This is similar to what happens with new cars. There is rarely a major improvement in new cars, but every year there are a host of new features. This is the engineering approach to device development.

Already available are defibrillators and pacemakers that measure pulmonary artery pressure in an effort to predict the development of acute decompensated heart failure. Another feature measures lung water in an effort to do the same thing. Predicting decompensated heart failure, it is hoped, will lead to earlier intervention to relieve congestion and avoid hospitalization for heart failure.

Battery life is also a key issue. As technology improves, batteries will need to be replaced less often. The next generation of defibrillators will also be better able to decide whether a shock needs to be delivered or not. Mary and Ed both would like to see the ability to predict who will need a defibrillator improve so that doctors can better focus this therapy on people most likely to suffer sudden death.

Assist Devices

A major redesign of the assist device will reduce its size even further and allow it to be completely implantable, making it more attractive to doctors and patients, with potential for decreasing the need for heart transplants. Having no line coming outside the body decreases the risk of infection. The devices will have a longer battery life, be less prone to develop blood clots, and have new features. A major change was the development of devices that provide continuous blood flow rather than blood flow in pulses. Continuous blood flow provides a continuous blood pressure that stays the same, which allows the device to be much smaller. Eventually there will be a research trial of heart transplantation versus a much improved left ventricular assist device. We are not there yet. These are all areas of active research, and it is impossible to predict when such devices might be available for use.

TREATMENT: BIOLOGICAL THERAPIES

Many people believe that biological therapies are the future of heart failure therapy. Biological therapy may involve the use of small proteins to either turn on or turn off genes, or the use of stem cells. As we understand more about the pathophysiology of heart failure, we will begin to understand where we might be able to turn on or off a gene to change the prognosis. For instance, we know that norepinephrine and angiotensin II are elevated in heart failure. What if we could turn off or decrease the function of these genes? Would this be of benefit? Nobody currently knows for sure. Stem cells will allow us, perhaps, to improve left ventricular function and limit left ventricular dilation. We may even be able to use stem cells to replace pacemakers, but these developments are all in the future.

Stem cells are cells that have the ability to develop into any kind of cell. It was once thought that we were born with all the heart cells we were ever going to get and that we had no ability to replace heart cells that die. This turns out not to be the case. Cardiac stem cells have been isolated from human hearts, and the heart seems to have the partial ability to repair itself using these cells. Cardiac stem cells are harvested from samples taken at heart biopsy and grown in a laboratory. They can then be reintroduced back into the heart. Stem cell therapies appear feasible, but there is still much research to be done into how to use them safely and successfully.

It is unclear right now what role stem cells play in the normal heart. Could there be a way to augment their normal function? Is there a way to increase their number? Is this something that we would even want to do? All these questions and more are yet to be answered but are being studied.

Cardiac stem cells avoid all the ethical issues involved in stem cells isolated from embryos. Investigators have also used bone marrow stem cells, which would normally grow to become such things as cartilage cells. Placed in the heart, these cells appear to repair damaged heart muscle by stimulating cardiac stem cells to multiply and mature into functioning heart cells. The future, then, will rely even more on understanding the basic biology of the human body.

SURGICAL ADVANCES: REMODELING

As described in chapter 8, much of the research in surgical therapy is directed at reversing the gradual remodeling that occurs in people with a weakened heart muscle. If the problem is that the left ventricle gradually assumes a spherical shape, the surgeon may be able to correct this. One operation under study involves trying to change the heart from a beach ball shape to more of a football shape by removing dead heart tissue. This operation, called *surgical ventricular restoration,* holds some promise. Preliminary results, however, are less exciting than originally thought.

Other surgeons have tried to constrain the heart from progressively dilating by using a girdlelike mesh device that is slipped around the heart. Struts have also been used to draw opposite walls of the left ventricle together to keep them from stretching out of shape.

SURGICAL ADVANCES: HEART TRANSPLANTATION

Most of the advance in human heart transplants is likely to come in the form of new drugs used to prevent rejection. *Xenotransplantation,* the transplantation of animal hearts into humans, may one day be possible. The most likely animal used would be a pig. The main problem that needs to be solved here is the transmission of retroviruses from animals to humans. The *human immunodeficiency virus* (HIV) is an example of a retrovirus initially found in chimpanzees and other monkeys that skipped into humans. Other such retroviruses exist, and xenotransplantation could allow one or more of these viruses to move from animals to humans. This would be an unacceptable price to pay for increasing the pool of donor hearts. Another reason pigs are more likely candidates, although they too harbor retroviruses, is that they can be grown to any size. In addition, we do not identify as closely with pigs, which we eat, as with chimpanzees. Preventing rejection will be a challenge in xenotransplants, too.

GENETICS AND PREVENTION

Better than any treatment would be the ability to prevent heart failure. As we learn more about the genetics of heart disease in general and heart failure in particular, we will begin to understand the interaction between our genes and the environment. Doctors know that cardiomyopathy is often inherited, but in the future we will understand how a genetic predisposition to cardiomyopathy is "turned on" to active disease by a specific environmental stimulus. For example, many people drink alcohol, but only a few develop a cardiomyopathy due to alcohol. There might be a gene or genes that put certain people at risk from the effects of alcohol and lead them to develop a dilated cardiomyopathy. Another example is myocarditis, which is a viral infection of the heart. In animals we know that certain strains of mice are susceptible to only certain strains of the same virus. In order to produce myocarditis, not only do you need the right genes, but the virus needs the right genes as well.

In the future, medicine will become more personalized. Genetics will be used to predict who will and who will not respond to certain therapies, much as oncologists are beginning to do in the treatment of cancer. An example is the detection of estrogen and progesterone receptors in breast cancer tumors. Tumors that produce estrogen or progesterone receptors are less likely to recur, less likely to be lethal, and more likely to respond to antiestrogen therapy. This commonly obtained test is used to guide therapy of women with breast cancer. We are at the very beginning of being able to use the genetic information we already have available for the benefit of heart patients. As we learn more and more, we will find new ways not only to treat heart failure but also to prevent the development of structural heart disease and heart failure.

ABOUT JOINING A THERAPY TRIAL

Making advances in the diagnosis and treatment of heart failure requires a discovery partnership between physicians interested in investigation and people with the condition. If you have heart failure or a cardiomyopathy, you may want to consider participating in clinical research. Your participation is essential in helping doctors discover and advance the science that will support new treatments for heart failure. Although you may not benefit directly, you will be helping future patients and those at risk for the syndrome.

The first thing to understand about a therapy trial is that if a researcher knew that a drug or device was better, she would not be doing research to show that it is. As a doctor interested in research, I may believe that the device or drug I am studying is better than what we use currently, but I cannot know that until I have done the research. Doctors and researchers do studies because we don't know the answer.

Good studies are done double blind, which means that neither the patient nor the doctor knows if the patient is getting the new drug or a placebo. We will not know which drug is better until the study is completed. Because most studies are placebo controlled, you may or may not get the new drug. This decision will be made randomly in a process much like flipping a coin. So again, while research improves the future for everyone with heart failure, it may not benefit you, should you decide to participate, either because you are one of the patients receiving placebo or standard therapy, or because the new therapy turns out not to be better than—or even as effective as—the standard therapy.

The decision to participate in medical research is highly personal. You must understand, however, what you are getting into. To participate, you will be asked to provide your *informed consent,* which is documented by your signature on a consent form. The key words here are "informed" and "consent." The second is easy to deal with. You must participate willingly and of your own volition. You should not feel coerced into participation.

The word "informed" is the more difficult. You should be informed about, and understand, everything written on the consent form you are asked to sign. Consent forms are written by the researcher and approved by a committee that is charged with oversight of all human experimentation at the institution where the research is being done. Such committees are called *institutional review boards,* or IRBs. If you do not understand something, ask for clarification. Make sure you know what is being asked of you, what tests will be done, and what benefits and risks you might experience. Only then will you be truly informed.

Part III

The CHALLENGES *of* LIVING *with* HEART FAILURE

12

Nutrition and Heart Failure

Samantha Heller, M.S., R.D., C.D.N.

Confessions of a nutritionist: As a child I loved salt. Scientists tell us that a taste for salt is an acquired taste, but my mother says I was born with one. When I was about seven years old, I used to go out in the field where a friend kept her horse and lick the horse's salt lick. Fortunately, he did not seem to mind sharing. Now that I am a nutritionist, of course, I have curbed my desire for salt by using other spices, herbs, lemon, vinegars, and other flavor enhancers. If pressed, I might say I still have a lingering fondness for salt. But I have learned to change an unhealthy habit, and that's why I know you can too.

In this chapter I explain how sodium, potassium, and good and bad fats affect heart failure. You will also find tips to kick start your heart-healthy lifestyle.

Starting a heart-healthy lifestyle will take some thoughtful planning. You will have to be open to making changes in your daily food choices and to trying new foods. Olive oil instead of butter can help keep your arteries from getting clogged and can reduce inflammation. Whole wheat toast with peanut butter in the morning in place of a doughnut or breakfast pastry can help you manage your weight and energy levels. And those spices and herbs instead of salt can help keep your sodium levels to a minimum, which is very important.

Food choices you make every day have a direct and profound impact on your heart health, energy level, immune system, and total health, because when food is digested, it gets broken down into molecules that become part of your cells and therefore part of your arteries, heart, brain, and other organs. Fruits, vegetables, whole grains, beans, and nuts provide your body with essential vitamins, minerals, fats, fiber, and plant compounds called *phytochemicals*. All these foods help the body fight disease, protect and repair damaged cells, and boost the cardiovascular, nervous, and immune systems. On the other hand, unhealthy foods like cheeseburgers, ice cream, butter, and fast foods are loaded with sodium and bad fats that increase the risk of cardiovascular and other diseases. The healthier your food choices, the healthier your body, and the better you feel.

Reaching and maintaining a healthy weight is an integral part of a heart-healthy lifestyle. Being overweight puts undue strain on your heart and increases your risk of developing or worsening existing diabetes, cancer, heart disease, and heart failure. Working with a registered dietitian can help you get started on a realistic healthy eating plan that works for you.

Be sure to weigh yourself every day at the same time and keep a record of your weight. If you have not significantly increased what you eat and yet you gain 3 to 5 pounds in a week—or even more weight in a shorter period—call your doctor immediately. The weight gain may be a signal that you are retaining too much fluid, which can put a strain on your heart and lungs. If your doctor has put you on a fluid restriction, monitor everything you drink (including soups, tea, coffee, fruit pops, ices, and diet sodas). Using a measuring cup will help you keep track of how much fluid you consume.

SODIUM

Sodium comes in many different forms and is hidden in surprising places. We usually think of sodium as table salt. Table salt is actually a combination of two minerals, sodium and chloride. Sodium is also in products like baking soda, baking powder, monosodium glutamate (MSG), disodium phosphate, garlic salt, sodium benzoate, and other additives.

Many of us love salt. We add it to just about everything: pasta, potatoes, eggs, vegetables, soups, fish, salsa, and tomato juice. I know someone who even salts her fruit. Everyone should limit sodium, but people with heart failure must be especially careful to do so. Most Americans eat well over the daily 2,300 mg of sodium recommended by the USDA *Dietary Guidelines for Americans 2005*. Some estimates put our intake of sodium at 4,000 mg a day or higher.

Sodium is necessary for a healthy body. But when we eat too much sodium, it can knock off the body's delicate balance of minerals and lead to problems in blood pressure and kidney function. In people with heart failure, eating too much salt can be more dangerous than it is for other people. When you have heart failure, your heart may not be pumping as efficiently as it should, and this can upset the fluid balance throughout the body. You may notice swelling in your ankles, feet, wrists, fingers, or abdomen, or a feeling of congestion or difficulty breathing after eating foods high in sodium (such as Chinese food, chips, and cheese). The reason is that sodium pulls water from surrounding tissues into the arteries. This increases the amount of fluid in the arteries, which raises blood pressure. The result is like having a garden hose (your arteries), turning the water on full blast (blood and water), and running it through a sprinkler's small pump (your heart). The extra fluid can strain the pumping action of the heart, lead to fluid buildup in the lungs, and cause swelling in your extremities. The increased blood pressure can damage your kidneys, arteries, and heart.

Dietary sodium is such a health concern that in June 2006, the American Medical Association released a report urging the Food and Drug Administration (FDA) to put warning labels on foods containing 480 mg or more per serving. For people with heart failure, heart disease, or high blood pressure, 1,500–2,000 mg per day or less of sodium is recommended. This means 1,500–2,000 mg of sodium for a whole day, not just one serving or meal. You may be surprised at how easy it is to eat that much salt at one meal. Just *one teaspoon* of table salt has about 2,400 mg of sodium.

Even if you have banned the salt shaker from the table and from cooking, you are likely getting more sodium in your diet than you realize. Over 75 percent of the sodium we eat is added to food during processing. Just two slices of pizza can contribute more than 1,500 mg of sodium. A single frozen dinner entrée may contain well over 3,000 mg of sodium (table 12.1).

Beware of Hidden Sodium

A patient of mine who has heart failure told me about food choices he made over the weekend. He and his wife had stopped at Wendy's for an afternoon snack, and he had ordered a Southwestern taco salad. Understandably, that seemed like a good choice for him, but that salad contains

Table 12.1. Range of Sodium Content for Selected Foods

Food group	*Serving size*	*Range of sodium content (mg)*
Breads	1 ounce	95–210
Frozen pizza	4 ounces	710–1,200
Frozen vegetables	1 cup	95–300
Salad dressing	2 tablespoons	110–400
Salsa	2 tablespoons	150–240
Soup (tomato)	8 ounces	700–1,100
Tomato juice	8 ounces	480–800

1,100 mg of sodium and 22 grams of fat! My patient was surprised and disappointed. "It didn't taste salty. And it was a salad, for goodness sakes!"

My taco salad eater is not alone in his confusion and frustration. One way to avoid running into hidden sodium is to go online to the Web site of most chain restaurants and get the nutrition information before you head out. In this case, Wendy's Mandarin Chicken Salad would have been a better choice, since it has only 480 mg of sodium and 2 grams of fat. If you do not use a computer, here are some safe bets: stay away from entrées and sides with high-sodium content or ingredients like cheese, salad dressings (except simple oil and vinegar), French fries, dipping sauces, bacon, and luncheon meats.

Because some sodium compounds are added to foods to increase shelf life, add texture, act as a preservative, or enhance flavor, the food may not *taste* salty. That does not mean that the sodium content is not high. Among the many foods that are unexpectedly high in sodium are sweets, breads, and cereals (see tables 12.1 and 12.2). Most prepared foods, like those from a restaurant, deli, or food bar, are high in sodium (table 12.2). A Starbucks vanilla Frappucino has 320 mg of sodium!

Nutrition information for chain restaurants can be found at the following Web sites:

Popeye's, www.popeyes.com/nutrition.pdf
Wendy's, www.wendys.com/food/NutritionLanding.jsp
McDonald's, www.mcdonalds.com/nutritionexchange/nutritionexchange.do
Starbucks, www.starbucks.com/retail/nutrition_comparison_popup.asp
KFC, www.kfc.com/nutrition

Pizza Hut, www.pizzahut.com/Nutrition.aspx
Diet Facts, www.dietfacts.com, lists nutrition information for the menus of several popular restaurants.

Going Low Sodium

Even if you love salt, as I used to, it takes only a few weeks to adjust your taste buds to a low-sodium diet. Pretty soon you will prefer the taste of lower sodium foods. Here's how to reduce your sodium intake:

1. Do not add salt to food at the table or in cooking. Instead, try these additions to perk up your meals:
   - Pepper, including black, lemon, and cayenne
   - Lemon and vinegars like balsamic, rice, and cider
   - Onions, garlic, scallions, and shallots
   - Dried or fresh herbs like rosemary, basil, dill, parsley, and sage
   - Low-sodium salsas
   - Exotic spices like curry, cumin, or chipotle peppers
2. Avoid these high-sodium condiments:
   - Spices with the word "salt" in the name, like onion salt or celery salt
   - Worcestershire sauce

Table 12.2. Sodium Content in Popular Restaurant Foods, Mall Foods, and Fast Foods

Food	*Sodium content (mg)*
Minestrone soup	610
Chicken Giardino, entrée	1,180
1 egg roll	460
Classic Reuben sandwich, 14 ounces	3,270
Fast food popcorn chicken, 6 ounces	1,050
Fast food apple pie, 1 slice	280
Fast food pecan pie, 1 slice, 4 ounces	510
Everything bagel, 4 ounces	710
Boston clam chowder, 8 ounces	1,060
Pepperoni pizza, 1 slice, 4 ounces	790
Fried chicken breast, 5½ ounces	1,120
French toast sticks (5), with syrup	460
Vanilla fudge brownie ice cream, ½ cup	100

Sources: Jacobsen, M.F., J.G. Hurley, Center for Science in the Public Interest. *Restaurant Confidential,* New York: Workman Publishing, 2002. For ice cream, see the manufacturer's Web site: www.haagendazs.com/segicd.do?productId=307

Soy sauce (even the "light soy" is high in sodium)
Horseradish
Barbeque sauce
Ketchup (use no-salt ketchup or make your own)
Dry packets of salad dressing and meat marinade mixes
Kosher and sea salt
Pickle relish
Seasoning blends
Premade sauces and mixes, which are likely to be high in sodium

3. When dining out, order your meal prepared without salt.
4. Look for fresh, unprocessed foods.

   Fresh vegetables, fruits, whole grains, and legumes are naturally low in sodium. Frozen produce is fine as long as it has no added sodium. To determine if there is added sodium, check the ingredients. (Bring your glasses or a magnifying glass, because the print is very small.) For example, if you buy a package of frozen broccoli, the ingredients should list only broccoli.
5. Read food labels.

   Below is a sample nutrition facts panel of a food label. Here's what to look for (or ignore) on these labels: Ignore the percentages on the righthand side. They can be confusing. What you really need to know is how many milligrams of sodium are contained in that particular food. Look specifically for the milligrams (mg) of sodium per serving. For example, consider the nutrition facts from the label on a box of macaroni and cheese:

   Nutrition Facts
   Serving Size 1 cup (228 g)
   Servings Per Container 2
   Total Fat 12 g
   Saturated Fat 3 g
   Trans Fat 3 g
   Cholesterol 30 mg
   Sodium 470 mg

   Note that one serving contains 470 mg of sodium. Now that you have this information, you can decide if it is worth spending 470 mg of the allotted 2,000 mg in a typical sodium-restricted diet on this particular food.

Remember to check the serving size. On this label, the serving is listed as 1 cup. If you eat 2 cups of the food, then you must double the amount of sodium, from 470 mg for one serving to 940 mg for two servings.

Most grocery stores sell many sodium-free canned foods, including vegetables, tomato products, soups, and sauces. Checking the nutrition label and reading the ingredients will tell you all you need to know about the sodium content of a product.

Here is the translation of some other information about sodium that appears on some labels (this information is from the Food and Drug Administration, *FDA Consumer*):

- Sodium free: less than 5 mg per serving
- Very low sodium: 35 mg or less per serving, or 35 mg or less per 50 g of the food
- Low sodium: 140 mg or less per serving, or 140 mg or less per 50 g of the food
- Salt-free: sodium-free
- Unsalted, without added salt, no salt added: no salt added during processing, and the food it resembles and for which it substitutes is normally processed with salt

6. Buy low-sodium or no-sodium versions of foods.
   Table 12.3 shows the difference between regular and low-sodium versions of several foods.

POTASSIUM

Potassium helps regulate your heartbeat and blood pressure, maintain your body's water balance, and facilitate neuromuscular function. The Institute of Medicine of the National Academies recommends we get 4,700 mg of potassium daily from food.

You may be on medications that increase or decrease your levels of potassium, or you may be taking some of each kind of medication. Since up to 90 percent of the element is excreted in the urine, if you are on diuretics, you may need to eat foods high in potassium, such as bananas or orange juice. But since you may also be on a heart medicine that causes you to retain potassium, be sure to discuss with your doctor whether you should or should not eat foods rich in potassium. A regis-

Table 12.3. Sodium Content, Regular versus Low-Sodium or No-Sodium Foods

Food	*Sodium content (mg)*
Baking powder, 1 teaspoon	488
Low-sodium baking powder, 1 teaspoon	4
Peanut butter, 2 tablespoons	147
Unsalted peanut butter, 2 tablespoons	5
Tomato puree, canned, 1 cup	998
No-sodium tomato purée, canned, 1 cup	70
Chicken noodle soup, ½ cup canned, condensed, made with water*	890
Low-sodium chicken noodle, 1 can*	120
Frozen broccoli, with salt, cooked, 1 cup	478
Frozen broccoli, no salt, cooked, 1 cup	20
Ham, 2 slices, about 2 ounces	730
Chicken breast, roasted, no skin, 3 ounces	64
Pretzels, salted, 10 twists	1,029
Pretzels, unsalted, 10 twists	173
Cheddar cheese, 1 ounce	176
Low-sodium cheddar cheese, 1 ounce	6
Corn muffin**	860
Whole wheat English muffin**	210

Source (except as noted below): USDA Nutrient Database Release 18[7]
*From manufacturer's Web site: Campbell's Soup www.campbellwellness.com
**From manufacturer's Web site: Dunkin' Donuts www.dunkindonuts.com/aboutus/nutrition

tered dietitian can help you plan what foods to include in your daily diet. Foods high and low in potassium and other selected nutrients are named at www.health.gov/dietaryguidelines (click on "Dietary Guidelines for Americans, 2005," and look for Appendix B-1). The DASH diet (Dietary Approaches to Stop Hypertension) is designed to help people adopt healthy eating habits and control high blood pressure (see www.nhlbi.nih.gov/health/public/heart/hbp/dash). It includes high-potassium foods such as vegetables and fruits.

GOOD FAT, BAD FAT

At the beginning of my lecture on fats at the New York University Medical Center or at a community program, I always ask, "Why is there fat on the planet? What is the purpose of fats?" One time a woman in the audience replied, "Fats are on this planet to torture us." That was not the answer I was looking for, but I could see her point. She was much relieved when I told her that fat not only helps food taste good, it is good for us, too. We must eat certain fats, like those that come from fish and walnuts, to survive. Our bodies use fats for these basic needs:

- energy
- absorbing vitamins A, D, E, and K
- forming cell membranes
- padding and protecting our organs and bones (imagine sitting down without any padding on your bottom)
- transmitting the taste of food
- making hormones such as testosterone
- forming vitamin D, bile, and other substances
- creating immunity and inflammation

Many of my patients have a real fear of eating any type of fat. They are concerned that guacamole will clog their arteries just the same as butter. But we need to eat fat to be healthy, and eating healthy fats does not necessarily make you fat. The secret to eating fats is distinguishing the good fats from the bad ones. The bad fats are trans fats and saturated fats. It is very important to limit saturated fats and avoid trans fats altogether. They can clog your arteries and increase your risk of chronic diseases. The good fats, the unsaturated fats, are essential for a healthy brain, nervous system, immune system, heart, and arteries. Keep in mind these fat basics when you're shopping and eating.

Saturated Fats and Trans Fats: The Bad Guys

Saturated fats are bad because they cause internal inflammation, raise bad cholesterol (low density lipoprotein, or LDL), impair artery function, and increase the risk of certain cancers. Saturated fats come primarily from animal sources such as meat, butter, cream, whole milk, ice cream, eggs, lard, and cheese. They are also found in tropical oils, such as coconut and palm, and cocoa butter. In the United States tropical oils are used mostly in processed foods, such as mass-produced cakes, cookies, candy, margarines, and candy bars. Here is an easy way to identify a saturated fat: it is solid at room temperature and for the most part comes from an animal. Check food labels to see how many grams of saturated fat are in a particular food.

Trans-fatty acids (also known as trans fats) are even worse for us than saturated fats. Trans-fatty acids raise bad cholesterol, reduce levels of good cholesterol (high density lipoprotein, or HDL), increase systemic inflammation, raise triglyceride levels, and increase the risk of diabetes.

Trans fats are the result of a process invented in 1902 in Germany called *hydrogenation,* which chemically alters liquid vegetable oils with heat and hydrogen to make them solid at room temperature and become more like a saturated fat. Hydrogenation is how corn oil, which is liquid at room temperature, is turned into a solid stick of margarine. Tub margarine is produced the same way, but with less hydrogenation. Hydrogenating fats also locks the fat in the food, so when you grab a handful of crackers or cookies out of the box, the oil does not drip out. Trans fats are an inexpensive way for food companies to keep the fat in cookies; deep-fry French fries, chicken, calamari, and doughnuts at high temperatures without burning them; keep crackers on the shelves longer; and make pie crusts flakier. The first and most popular result of hydrogenation was Crisco vegetable shortening, introduced by Procter and Gamble in 1911.

How Much Is Too Much?

According to the American Heart Association (AHA), you may consume between 16 and 20 grams (g) of saturated fat a day. The amount you may eat depends on your activity level and caloric intake. The easiest way to lower saturated fat is to choose low-fat or nonfat animal foods such as milk, cheese, cottage cheese, or yogurt, which have most or all of the bad fat removed.

The types of animal foods you can have every day include skinless white meat of poultry like chicken and turkey (the dark meat such as in drumsticks has much more saturated fat than the white meat), swimming fish (shellfish are high in cholesterol), egg whites, and low-fat or nonfat dairy products. Limit your consumption of animal foods that are *not* low-fat or nonfat to special occasions. When a holiday or birthday party is on the calendar, you can look forward to having reasonable portions of a food high in saturated fat, like 3 to 4 ounces of steak, half a cup of ice cream, or a small slice of Aunt Susi's famous coconut cream pie.

As far as trans fats, no acceptable or safe amount has been determined by the FDA. The Nurses' Health Study of 80,000 women, reported in the British medical journal the *Lancet*, found that 50 percent were more likely to develop heart disease if 3 percent of their daily calories came from trans fats than if 1 percent of their calories came from trans fats. For an average intake of 2,000 calories a day, 3 percent adds up to only about 7 grams of trans fat, the amount in one fast food croissant or a doughnut. A study in the *New England Journal of Medicine* reported that removing trans fats from the industrial food supply could prevent tens of thousands of heart attacks and cardiac deaths each year in the United States.

Here are some tips to help you avoid the trans, or hydrogenated, fats that are found in many store-bought and restaurant-prepared foods: First, check the nutrition facts panel found on packaged foods. Look for the number of trans fats grams. Then read the ingredients. If the words "partially hydrogenated" or "hydrogenated" appear in the ingredient list, then that product *does* contain trans fats. Do not be confused if the label lists 0 g of trans fats but the word "hydrogenated" still appears in the list of ingredients. The FDA allows the label to say 0 g of trans fats if a product contains less than 0.5 grams of trans fats per serving. However, if you eat more than one serving of that food, the trans fats can start adding up. The words "partially hydrogenated" and "hydrogenated" are the real clues.

By reducing the trans fats and saturated fats in your diet, you will lower your risk of heart disease and other chronic diseases. Replace saturated and trans fats with healthy fats. Use olive oil instead of butter; buy trans fat-free crackers, baked goods, frozen foods, and other grocery items; and skip the deep-fried foods in restaurants.

Cholesterol: The Bad and the Good Guy

Cholesterol is one of those lipids our bodies need for survival. Cholesterol is so necessary for a healthy body that it is manufactured in our liver. Our bodies use it to make hormones, such as testosterone and estrogen, and vitamin D, and it is also an important part of our cell membranes. Yet too much circulating cholesterol in our bloodstream can result in plaque buildup in our arteries, causing heart disease.

Our liver is capable of making all the cholesterol we need. Cholesterol is also found in the foods we eat that come from animals, like milk, cheese, beef, and ham. Genetics plays a significant role in how much cholesterol the body makes. Some people suffer no harm from eating foods rich in cholesterol, while others are harmed by very little. Your cholesterol level is easily measured by a blood test. These levels change. You may have had low to average cholesterol for most of your life before at some point, your cholesterol level jumps too high. Cholesterol is not the same thing as saturated fat, but the two are almost always found together.

Even if you have low cholesterol, are at a healthy weight, and exercise, you still need to limit the amount of saturated fat you eat. The inflammation that saturated fat causes and the rise in bad cholesterol happens in everyone's body. A number of my patients with normal cholesterol levels exercised regularly and therefore thought they could eat anything they wanted. They had a very unpleasant reminder about the importance of diet when they found themselves in the ER with chest pain.

While genetics plays an important role in how much and how well our bodies process cholesterol, how we eat has a significant impact on our risk for cardiovascular disease.

The Egg Question

The National Heart, Lung and Blood Institute (NHLBI) recommends we eat only 200 mg of cholesterol per day. One egg yolk contains about 210 mg of cholesterol. This is more than we should have in a whole day. The egg whites do not contain cholesterol or saturated fat. Although it is okay to eat an egg yolk once in a while, remember that you will be eating other foods during the day that contain cholesterol, and it can add up. The NHLBI recommends you have two or fewer yolks per week, including yolks in baked goods and in cooked or processed foods.

The Good Fats: Unsaturated

In addition to bad fats, foods also contain unsaturated fats that are good for you and necessary for a healthy body. These healthy fats help you fight cardiovascular and other diseases and are important for the health of your immune, neurological, and cardiovascular systems. Unsaturated fats are found in plants, nuts, and fish and are liquid at room temperature. They are called *mono*unsaturated fats and *poly*unsaturated fats. The polyunsaturated fats include the very healthy omega-3 fatty acids. Recent evidence suggests that omega-3 fatty acids may have a role in the prevention and treatment of cardiovascular disease, including fatal heart attacks, as well as a range of other diseases, including diabetes mellitus, breast cancer, arthritis, other inflammatory diseases, Alzheimer's, lung disease, and autoimmune disorders. Omega-3 fatty acids are found in fish and fish oils, canola oil, leafy vegetables, flaxseed oil, ground flaxseed, walnuts, and soybeans.

Many foods contain a combination of different forms of fats. Peanut butter, for example, is primarily a monounsaturated fat, but it also has polyunsaturated fats and even a little saturated fat. This little bit of saturated fat is acceptable since most of the fat in the peanut oil is healthy unsaturated fat. Nuts and nut butters, like peanut, almond, and cashew, are good for us. But you have to read the labels. Buy nut butters that do not have added salt or sugar. Many commercial peanut butters contain partially hydrogenated oils to keep the oil from separating from the nut solids. You are better off with the "natural" nut butters, the ones that have the oil on the top. You will have to stir the butter up to mix the oils with the nuts (it is messy, so do this in the sink). Once they are mixed, keep the nut butter in the refrigerator and they won't reseparate. Some people pour the oil off, thinking the fat is bad for them, but the unsaturated fats in nuts are good fats, so *do not* pour them off. If you live near a health food store that grinds fresh nut butters, that's even better.

A diet with a variety of foods ensures that you are getting both mono- and polyunsaturated oils.

What's the Bottom Line?

Eating trans fats, saturated fats, and cholesterol can increase your risk for heart disease, stroke, obesity, diabetes, and cancer. These fats come from animals and from tropical oils and are often found in processed foods.

Polyunsaturated and monounsaturated fats come primarily from plant sources and fish and do not raise serum cholesterol levels or increase your risk for disease. These healthy oils contain antioxidants and additional compounds that fight disease. Poly- and monounsaturated oils include olive, canola, peanut, sesame, walnut, flaxseed, grapeseed, and safflower.

I must add a cautionary note here, which is that *all fats* contain approximately the same amount of calories. A tablespoon of butter, a saturated fat, has about the same number of calories (around 100) as a tablespoon of olive oil, an unsaturated fat. To avoid gaining weight, use even healthy fats moderately.

The benefits of a heart-healthy lifestyle are tremendous. Within about two weeks of starting to eat the heart-healthy way, you will begin to feel healthier and more energetic. Keep in mind, however, that lifestyle changes can be difficult. You may stumble periodically and feel frustrated at times, but don't give up. These feelings are a normal part of changing old habits and learning new ones. Look for the healthiest food choice at each meal and plan ahead. If you know you have a vacation or party coming up, think in advance about what food choices you will make on those occasions. Bring healthy foods with you when you travel or are going to have a long day away from home.

Call restaurants ahead of time and discuss their menu. A good time to call a restaurant to speak with the chef or manager is in the late afternoon, before the dinner rush. When ordering, do not be afraid to ask how foods are prepared, and ask to have the chef prepare your food without salt, cream, butter, or cheese. Order your selections grilled, baked, broiled, or steamed. These days restaurants are used to people with special dietary needs, so there is no reason to feel shy about making your needs known.

HEART-HEALTHY SHOPPING LISTS AND MEAL SUGGESTIONS

This list of foods will help get you started on a heart-healthy lifestyle. I encourage you to try new foods. Include a variety of foods so you can benefit from all the health-promoting nutrients nature has to offer.

Shopping Lists

Carbohydrates

Choose whole grains.

Whole grain bread
Whole wheat pasta
Oatmeal
100 percent whole grain ready-to-eat cereals
Whole grain crackers, pretzels (no salt)
Whole grain tortillas
Quinoa
Brown and wild rices
Soy crisps
Rice cakes
Baked chips
Whole grain pancake mix
Frozen, trans fat-free, whole grain waffles
Whole grain English muffins
Whole wheat bagels
No-fat popped corn

Proteins and Fats

Skinless chicken or turkey white meat
Egg whites, egg beaters
Soy foods: tofu, edamame, soy milk, soy nuts, soy cheese
Legumes: kidney beans, chick peas, black-eyed peas, lentils, split peas, white beans, pink beans, red beans, black beans, and navy beans (hint: rinse canned beans to reduce the amount of sodium)
Hummus
Nonfat or 1 percent milk
Nonfat or low-fat cheese, yogurt, cottage cheese, sour cream, cream cheese
Nonfat or low-fat frozen yogurt, ice cream
Olive, canola (expeller pressed, organic), sesame, peanut, walnut oils
Peanut, almond, cashew butters ("natural")
Nuts (roasted, unsalted), seeds (pumpkin, sunflower)

Fish

Fish are an excellent source of lean protein and healthy omega-3 fats. To get a good dose of omega-3 fats in your diet, the AHA recommends eating fish like mackerel, lake trout, herring, sardines, and salmon at least two times a week.

Some fish are high in mercury. *Do not eat white albacore tuna, shark, swordfish, king mackerel, or tile fish.* Fish that have lower mercury levels tend to be smaller fish like salmon, sole, tilapia, orange roughy, catfish, pollack, and sardines. Check the Environmental Protection Agency and the FDA's Web sites for updates and local advisories about the safety of local catch. Eating cooked shellfish (never raw) is acceptable once in a while, but shellfish tend to be high in cholesterol.

Miscellaneous

Low-sodium nonfat soups
Vegetarian chili
Low-sodium, low-fat, healthy frozen entrées
Low-sodium tomato sauce
Low-sodium salsa and bean dips
Dark chocolate (70 percent or more cocoa)
All-fruit popsicles and bars

Fruits and Vegetables

Any and all you like (and even some you don't)
Fresh or frozen (no salt added)
Canned (no sodium)

Beverages

Limit amounts of juices and some other beverages you drink because they can pack more calories in a day than people expect. As long as your doctor approves, however, you can consume many of the so-called all-day beverages to stay hydrated. One all-day beverage idea is a spritzer with half juice and half sparkling or plain spring water. Keep in mind that adults should consume about 2 to 3 servings of fruit a day and that a 6-ounce glass of 100 percent juice counts as one fruit.

Note that if your doctor has advised you to limit beverages, you need to follow your doctor's advice. A common fluid restriction is 2 liters (or about 70 ounces) of fluid a day. If you don't have any restrictions on how much you can drink, you might consider any of thesc all-day beverages:

Coffee (decaf or regular)
Teas
Diet drinks
Water or flavored waters
Seltzer or flavored seltzers
Nonfat milk or soy milk
Nonfat hot chocolate (skip the whip)

Meal Suggestions

Below you will find individual meal suggestions. Feel free to embellish them with extra vegetables, fruits, or herbs and spices. You can mix and match and have a "lunch" meal for breakfast or vice versa. I happen to like tofu and vegetables for breakfast. In China a common morning meal is vegetables, fish, and rice. It all depends on what you like and what is available to you.

Breakfast

Whole grain cereal (hot or cold), nonfat milk, walnuts, and ¾ cup berries or half a banana
Egg white omelet with spinach and mushrooms, and whole wheat toast
Multigrain bagel with low-fat cream cheese, tofu cream cheese, or peanut butter

Lunch

Peanut butter and jelly sandwich on whole grain bread
Grilled vegetable wrap, whole wheat tortilla, chicken breast
Salad, *lots* of vegetables, with chick peas, tuna, tofu, or turkey
Nonfat grilled cheese with tomato, whole wheat bread
Hummus, whole wheat pita, vegetables
Low-sodium vegetarian chili
Veggie burger

Tuna fish (chunk light) made with low-fat mayonnaise or hummus, chopped celery, peppers, and onions

Snacks

Handful of unsalted nuts
Nonfat plain yogurt with cereal or trail mix (nonfat fruit yogurt is okay but has more calories; buy plain and add your own fruit)
Low-fat cottage cheese and mini rice cakes
Low-fat cheddar cheese and apple
Hummus or baba ganouj and cut-up vegetables
Almond butter and whole grain crackers
Steamed vegetable dumplings (no soy sauce)

Dinner

Have all sauces on the side so that you can control the amount you use.

Strips of grilled chicken breast and broccoli over whole wheat pasta, with low-sodium sauce of your choice
White beans with roasted garlic, broccoli rabe, and broiled Portobello mushrooms
Low-sodium, low-fat frozen entrées, with a salad or extra vegetables
Turkey chili with nonfat sour cream, baked no-salt chips, salad
Baked chicken with a vegetable of your choice and wild rice
Mixed vegetable and tofu stir fry, brown rice, low-sodium teriyaki sauce (Sam Heller's favorite)
Rockfish, catfish, or orange roughy in lemon or white wine sauce, asparagus, salad (Mary Knudson's favorite)
Grilled salmon brushed with olive oil, spinach salad, fruit (Ed Kasper's favorite)

Desserts

The serving size for frozen desserts is half a cup.

All-fruit sorbet
Nonfat frozen yogurt
1 cup fruit salad
Nonfat pudding snacks (192 mg of sodium)

Toffuti Chocolate Fudge Treats (frozen)
Small piece dark chocolate
Two 100 percent whole grain Fig Newtons

Eating Out

Ask that your food be prepared without salt, butter, cheese, or cream. Order all sauces on the side.

Italian

Eggplant parmesan without the cheese (but keep in mind that restaurant tomato sauce is high in sodium), whole grain garlic bread made with olive oil
Pizza (whole wheat crust if you can find it), vegetables, no cheese or nonfat mozzarella or soy cheese
Whole wheat pasta primavera (most restaurants do not have whole wheat pasta, but it is worth a try)

Mexican

Vegetable and chicken burrito, guacamole (skip sour cream and cheese), low-sodium refried beans made with canola oil
Spinach, mushroom, poblano peppers, grilled onion quesadilla (no cheese)

Indian

Curried mixed vegetables and lentils
Chicken tandoori

Chinese

Steamed chicken and mixed vegetables, brown rice, side of sauce

American

Fresh fish, baked or grilled
Chick peas, sun-dried tomatoes, fresh sprouts, and grilled chicken on a bed of fresh baby spinach
Vegetarian burger with salad

Healthy Eating Quick Points

Keep track of your daily sodium intake. The *Dietary Guidelines for Americans* allow 2,300 mg per day. Your doctor may advise you to consume less sodium than that. These steps also help you avoid health problems:

- **Weigh yourself at the same time every day.**
- **Discuss your potassium needs with your doctor.**
- **Read nutrition facts panels (food labels) and ingredients lists:**
  milligrams (mg) of sodium
  grams (g) of saturated fat
  grams (g) of trans fats
  hydrogenated or partially hydrogenated
- **Choose low- or nonfat animal foods.**
- **Avoid all trans fats.**
- **Reduce amount of high-fat animal foods (cheese, ice cream, beef, luncheon meats, whole milk, and so on).**
- **Use healthy plant oils.**
- **Eat fish at least once a week.**
- **Eat a variety of fruits and vegetables every day.**
- **Plan ahead.**
- **Try new foods and be creative.**

MYTH BUSTERS

Newspapers, magazines, TV, and radio sometimes report the latest medical research and dietary recommendations without including important context, or they report the findings in a confusing way. Here are some food myths that have been perpetuated and that are in need of being "busted."

"Carbohydrates will make you fat."

A phobia about carbohydrates ("carbophobia") generated by fad diet books in the 1990s and into the following century caused all sorts of confusion. Simply stated, carbohydrates are *good* for you and very necessary for a healthy body. All carbohydrates get broken down in the body to sugar, also known as glucose. Glucose is the primary and preferred source of fuel for your brain and working muscles. This sugar provides the body with the energy it needs to function. Carbohydrates include starches like bread, pasta, crackers, rolls, and cereals. They are also found in beans, fruits, vegetables, and dairy products like milk (the lactose in milk is a form of sugar).

The kind of carbs you eat makes the difference. Look for the whole grain versions of your favorite carbs, like whole wheat pasta, whole grain cereals (oatmeal, shredded wheat), bread, crackers, and even oatmeal cookies (made without butter). Whole grains such as whole wheat, oats, barley, quinoa, kasha, and brown and wild rices have all their original nutrients, fiber, vitamins, and minerals and offer a more consistent release of energy during the day than candy and other sugary food.

Avoid white starchy foods like white bread and pasta, pretzels, crackers, and foods high in sugar like soda, cookies, cakes and other sweets, cereals that are not whole grain, and white rice. These foods tend to lead to energy crashes, are high in calories, and when consumed regularly may increase the risk for obesity, cardiovascular disease, and diabetes.

"All fats are bad."

This nutrition myth has shown some serious staying power. We've discussed how including good fats in your diet is necessary for a healthy cardiovascular, immune, and central nervous system. Go ahead, have some guacamole, peanut butter, or olive oil. Just don't chow down big portions, because even though these plant oils are good for you, they are also high in calories.

"Just a little bit won't make a difference."

Unfortunately, "a little bit" of a lot of things can add up daily. Be thoughtful when you make exceptions to your healthy diet and never go overboard. If you have heart failure and retain fluid, one high-sodium meal (Mexican food, pepperoni pizza) can put you at risk for a trip to the emergency room. If on a special occasion you want some cake or a piece of steak or even some Chinese food, be sure to have small portions of these foods. For example, have a 3- to 4-ounce portion of steak instead of a 16-ounce piece of meat. Order Chinese food steamed with brown rice and with sauce on the side. Eat slowly and savor the flavor and the moment.

"It's 'all natural,' so it must be good for me."

Arsenic is all natural, but eating it is not good for you. The phrase "all natural" implies that the product is healthy for you, and many of us are seduced into believing that is true. An "all natural" product and even some organic products may be high in sodium, saturated fat, refined sugars, or calories. Read the nutrition facts panel and the ingredients list carefully to determine if a food or product is something you want to consume.

SUPPLEMENTS AND HEART FAILURE

Always ask your doctor before taking any supplements or herbs, because they may interact with your medications. If you do use a supplement, ask if you need to take it at a different time from your medications.

A Multivitamin

When you have heart failure, your body may need a little extra boost of certain vitamins, minerals, or other compounds. For many people, a daily multivitamin is a good idea. Ask your doctor if taking one is right for you.

Vitamin D

Recent studies have suggested that heart failure patients tend to be deficient in vitamin D and that supplementation may help improve heart function and protect the heart by reducing circulating inflammatory compounds. Research is still ongoing, however, and the appropriate dosages have yet to be determined. The current recommendation for adults is 400–600 IU (international units) of vitamin D each day, or 10–15 mcg (micrograms) of vitamin D each day, with the upper tolerable limit (UL) set at 2,000 IU (50 mcg). Some experts are suggesting the UL be set as high as 10,000 IU (250 mcg). For people with heart failure, researchers recommend a daily oral dose of 50–100 mcg (2,000–4,000 IU) vitamin D. Taking too much, however, can lead to vitamin D toxicity, so for now it is best for most people to stick with the current recommendation of 400–600 IU (10–15 mcg) per day. Ask your doctor about the appropriate dose for you.

Many people should be getting more vitamin D in their diets. Vitamin D is found in oily fish such as mackerel, sardines, and salmon; fortified ready-to-eat cereals; and milk. We also get vitamin D from exposing our skin to sunlight, and it is found in most multivitamin pills. This vitamin is important for a healthy immune system, strong bones, and calcium absorption.

Magnesium

Magnesium is used in more than 300 biochemical reactions in the body, including proper muscle, nerve, and heart function; protein synthesis; and energy metabolism. The National Institutes of Health reports that most Americans are not getting enough magnesium in their diets. Patients with heart failure may be particularly at risk for low magnesium levels due to poor food intake, medications, and other complications associated with heart failure.

The best way to get adequate magnesium is with whole foods. Excellent sources include avocados, almonds, cashews, pumpkin seeds, spinach, oats, and whole grain cereals. You might also need a supplement of magnesium or a multivitamin that contains magnesium. The current Recommended Dietary Allowance (RDA) for magnesium is 420 mg for men over age 31, and 320 mg for women over age 31.

Coenzyme Q10

Coenzyme Q10 (CoQ10) has become a popular supplement in recent years. It is a compound found in many foods, including soy, canola oils, sardines, chicken, and peanuts. CoQ10 is used in energy production in the body, is an antioxidant, and is involved in other biological processes, including muscle contraction and immune system functions.

Though not conclusive, scientific research suggests that supplementing with CoQ10 may benefit people with heart disease and those with heart failure. Results from studies indicate that CoQ10 supplementation may help improve heart muscle and blood vessel function, protect the heart muscle during and after cardiac surgery, reduce sore muscles associated with cholesterol-lowering medications, and replenish low levels of

CoQ10 caused by the presence of heart disease, heart failure, or statin drugs. Cardiologists differ in their opinion about whether supplementing with CoQ10 is helpful for patients with heart failure.

Coenzyme Q10 supplements are found in vitamin and health food stores, grocery stores, and drug stores. Regrettably, they tend to be expensive. If you and your doctor decide that you should be taking CoQ10, be sure to take it with a meal containing some fat (like olive oil, almond butter, salad dressing) to enhance absorption. Discuss the dosage with your doctor.

13

Exercise

How Much and What Kind?

You may want to think of yourself as an athlete in training, because if you've been diagnosed with heart failure, you need to condition your body for the rest of your life. Exercising is an essential part of living well with heart failure. If you develop the mindset, as athletes do, that conditioning your body is part of your daily responsibility, you may find it easier to follow through with regular exercise.

That's not to promise that exercising six days a week, week after week after week, is easy. It's not for me. I (Mary) need all the help I can get, and I still sometimes cop out. But then I renew my commitment to faithfully execute my exercise routine. I've worked to create an environment—including getting a trainer, the right exercise equipment, and more focus and discipline—to help me stick with my exercise program. You may be able to exercise in a more informal way on your own or with an exercise buddy. We each have to find a system that works for us. We'll discuss how to do that in this chapter. But before you or I commit to exercising, we must first understand why we need to do it.

WHY EXERCISE?

To keep from turning into a statue; gain more freedom of movement; ease our heart's workload; strengthen our core body, legs, arms, heart, and lungs; and become more active, we need to exercise. A main symptom of heart failure is an inability to exercise for long, or even to do normal activities such as walking or bathing without feeling fatigued or short of breath. Heart failure doesn't just affect your heart. It also affects many of the muscles in your body, and muscle weakness is often most noticeable in your legs.

At least three things contribute to your muscle weakness: As your heart labors to send oxygen to your body, your skeletal muscles receive less oxygen, certain damaging chemical changes occur, and using the muscles makes them tire easily. Your symptoms of heart failure—your general fatigue, shortness of breath, and muscle fatigue—often lead to your becoming less active. I spoke about this with Kerry J. Stewart, Ed.D., director of clinical and research exercise physiology, Johns Hopkins University School of Medicine. "The main benefits of exercise in patients with heart failure are to improve the function of the muscles so that they are better able to use the oxygen carried by the blood, thereby decreasing the demand for more blood from the heart," he explained. Dr. Stewart works with heart patients and is a co-author of guidelines for resistance training adopted in 2007 by the American Heart Association (AHA). "By staying active," he said, "the muscles will also better retain their tone and avoid atrophy, thereby preventing or delaying disability. The goal is to avoid the cycle of disability that is so common when patients with heart failure are very sedentary."

Part of my plan to be active was to get a trainer. I share a trainer with the 2008 U.S. Olympic Soccer Team. Yes, really. I am so proud of him. I met him in 2006, the same way anyone could, going to his place of work as a client. Randy Rocha is director of sports medicine for Metro Orthopedics and Sports Therapy Centers in two Maryland locations. He is a certified athletic trainer and strength and conditioning coach for D.C. United professional men's and youth soccer teams, and he is a trainer for Washington Freedom professional women's soccer team. He was just what I was looking for: a strength and conditioning coach. In addition to heart failure, I had developed an unrelated difficulty walking any distance. So I had double incentive to strengthen my body.

Through his work at the sports therapy center, Randy has seen a wide range of men and women of all ages with movement problems. He explains that with inactivity, as can happen when people first develop heart failure or have moderate to severe heart failure, muscle tightening and muscle atrophy set in. "You atrophy so much that you don't have the strength to get from point A to point B. So of course you're going to be sore all the time. Not only is everything atrophying; everything's tightening up, and it's slowly getting tighter and tighter." Then when you try to get up from a chair or off the toilet or walk up stairs or even walk on a flat surface, your shrunken muscles can't meet the demands. So you may find yourself hobbling along, stopping to rest your hands on the back of a chair or to lean against a wall. Not the shape you want to be in? Regular stretching and strengthening exercises will help you get up more naturally and walk more normally, with better posture, for longer periods.

Most heart failure occurs in people who are over 55, so aside from your heart failure, you may have also gotten out of shape, be overweight, and have some arthritis, diabetes, or other medical problems. Like me, you have multiple reasons to exercise. When you plan your exercise routine, be sure to treat your heart failure, but also take care of your whole body's needs. Besides the ability to be more active and do more things, benefits from exercising include lower blood pressure and improved ability of the blood vessels to expand and contract.

HOW TO EXERCISE

Heart failure is different in each of us—the cause, the extent of its effect on your heart and all of your body's muscles, how well you can keep it from progressing, or whether you completely get over it. What kind and how much exercise you do should be tailored to your individual physical situation. It is very important to discuss exercise with the doctor who is treating you for heart failure. Your doctor can tell you if it is not safe for you to exercise at all. Most patients with heart failure, though, do benefit from exercise. For most of us, it is not only safe to exercise, it is healthy.

Do not settle for advice that you should walk 20 or 30 minutes a day. Walking is a great exercise. But most of us should not stop there. Ask if there is any specific medical reason that prevents you from doing aerobic or resistance exercises. Resistance exercising, also known as strength training, has gained the approval of the AHA for most heart patients. But check first. The AHA guidelines, called *Absolute and Relative Contraindications to Resistance Training*, are reproduced in the sidebar that follows. Take these guidelines to your doctor and ask if you have any of the conditions listed under "Absolute" that would prohibit you from doing resistance exercises. If you have a condition listed under "Relative," discuss your ability to do resistance exercises with your doctor before starting an exercise program.

Some doctors know more about exercise than others. Be sure your doctor knows what you are referring to when you ask about resistance training. What we mean by resistance training is low to moderate exercise using elastic therabands, machine weights, or free weights that are just the amount of weight you can handle as determined by an exercise specialist. We're not talking about lying on your back or standing in a crouched position and then straining maximally to lift handheld dumbbells or barbells over your head. You want to avoid heavy straining. Again, be sure your doctor understands what you mean when you ask if you can do resistance exercises.

Once you know what you do and don't have wrong medically, you

---

Absolute and Relative Contraindications to Resistance Training

Absolute Contraindications

If you have any of these conditions, do not do resistance exercises:

- **Unstable (active) coronary heart disease (having chest pain at rest or with minimal exertion)**
- **Decompensated heart failure (having severe symptoms of heart failure such as shortness of breath, fatigue, and fluid retention even though you are being treated for heart failure)**
- **Uncontrolled arrhythmias**
- **Severe pulmonary hypertension (mean pulmonary arterial pressure > 55 mmHg)**
- **Severe and symptomatic aortic stenosis**
- **Acute myocarditis, endocarditis, or pericarditis**
- **Uncontrolled high blood pressure (> 180/110 mmHg; do not do resistance exercise until you get more treatment and your blood pressure falls below 160/100)**
- **Aortic dissection**
- **Marfan syndrome**
- **Active proliferative retinopathy or moderate or worse nonproliferative diabetic retinopathy (avoid high-intensity resistance training, 80% to 100% of 1-RM [one repetition maximum])**

Relative Contraindications

If you have any of these conditions, consult a doctor before participating in resistance exercise:

- **Major risk factors for coronary heart disease (diabetes, smoking, high blood pressure, high cholesterol)**
- **Diabetes at any age (if diabetes is controlled, resistance exercise is okay and even recommended by the American Diabetes Association)**
- **Uncontrolled high blood pressure ($\geq 160/\geq 100$ mmHg; you can exercise if your blood pressure is below this level, even while taking medications to control blood pressure)**
- **Low functional capacity (< 4 METs [metabolic equivalent tasks]; METs are a measurement of exercise capacity)**
- **Musculoskeletal limitations (if the problem is so severe that it severely limits walking)**
- **Implanted pacemaker or defibrillator**

Source:* American Heart Association Science Advisory, *Resistance Exercise in Individuals with and without Cardiovascular Disease: 2007 Update.

can find an exercise specialist to get you started in an exercise program tailored for you. If you have an ongoing problem with your heart, it is wise to begin your exercise program while supervised by someone experienced in working with heart patients. A cardiac rehabilitation program will communicate with your doctor to be sure that the exercise program developed for you is based on your medical history, medications you take, and any implanted devices you have, such as a pacemaker or defibrillator. You can have your heart monitored as you exercise, and you'll also get advice on lifestyle changes like stopping smoking and eating a healthy diet with limited salt, no trans fats, and limited saturated fats (see chapter 12). It is best to get advice from the experts rather than trying anything on your own. Find out what your doctor can do to get you professional advice and supervision in exercise and nutrition.

If you have reached a point of progress in which your heart is now functioning with a normal ejection fraction and you are not having symptoms of heart failure, you may choose instead to check out a sports therapy center, which will probably have clients of a wider age range, who are there for a variety of reasons. Or you may decide to meet one on one with a physical therapist or certified trainer. Find the environment that projects an energy and comfort level that works for you. You'll find it helpful to get started with an expert showing you what exercises to do, how to do them, and how much rest to take between exercise sets before eventually continuing your workouts on your own, at a facility or at home.

Whatever setting you choose, be sure that a therapist first tests you to determine your levels of strength and movement and then watches as you do prescribed exercises. If your therapist is working with so many people that he does not watch how you do your exercises, find another program. It is very important to learn to do exercises correctly to avoid hurting yourself and to get the most benefit from them.

These are some basic questions to ask a therapist or trainer:

- What exercises should I do?
- In what order should I do them?
- How long should each exercise last? (How many repetitions?)
- How frequently should I do each exercise? (More than once a day? Every day? Two or three days a week?)
- How long do I need to rest between exercises or between exercise sessions? (The right workout-rest ratio is important for people with active heart failure. Start with short exercises and progress as you get stronger.)
- How will I know when to progress to more intensity with my exercises? (When should I increase weight or number of repetitions?)

TYPES OF EXERCISE

If your doctor says you are healthy enough to exercise and have no particular exercise restrictions, choose a combination of these three types:

1. *Stretching exercises* will isolate individual muscles, lengthen them, and keep them and your joints flexible.
2. *Aerobic exercise,* also called *cardiovascular exercise,* such as biking or walking will build the heart's endurance and improve muscle function in your legs and arms, depending on the exercise you do.

3. *Resistance exercises or strength training* can strengthen muscles throughout your body, increase muscle endurance, and improve balance and posture. Increasing muscle endurance can improve the body's ability to burn fat throughout the day.

In addition, if you are strong enough, *balance exercises,* such as standing on a balance board or wobble board, will improve your body's awareness in space. If you do these balancing exercises, you must place your board very close to a railing or other sturdy structure that you can grip to keep from falling. You should also place the board on a rubber mat or rubber floor to help keep the board from slipping.

You can also do balance exercises without using a balance board or wobble board. Try standing on one foot, standing on one or both feet with your eyes closed (but hold on to something or have someone stand next to you if you close your eyes), sit on top of a theraball, or practice marching, lifting one leg at a time, eyes open, near something sturdy you can grab if you need to.

Stretching Exercises

Stretching your calf muscles in your lower leg, your quadriceps (the major muscles in the front of the thigh), and hamstrings (in the back of the thigh) is important for walking well and not tiring easily. Stretching the muscles surrounding the hips—glutes, hamstrings, and iliotibial band—can help reduce back pain and improve posture.

Aerobic (Cardiovascular) Exercise

Examples of aerobic exercise are biking outdoors or riding a stationary bike, walking outdoors or on a treadmill, running or jogging, and using an elliptical trainer. These exercises, which you'll spend the most time doing, get your heart rate up. They also burn fat and help you lose weight. A recent study found that aerobic exercise helps remodel an enlarged left ventricle to a more normal size.

Walking 20 to 30 minutes a day is a great aerobic exercise if you can manage it. You may want to have a regular time each day to walk outside with a friend. Or you could walk for 20 minutes just going through the aisles of a large supermarket, though you probably would not be able to go at the pace recommended for this heart-healthy exercise without the risk of crashing into another cart or display of apples. But walking in a grocery store is a good way to get started. If you need some support when you walk, a grocery cart acts as a great walker on wheels.

To get around other types of stores, you may find it helpful to take with you a rolling cart with a basket that you can put packages in as you shop. The cart frees you from carrying bulky or heavy items and, again, serves the purpose of a walker, something to lean on as you go from your car into the store and back to the car. You can order these carts through the Internet. But if you can get along without a walking aid, do. My trainer, Randy, cautions that continual use of a walking aid of any kind, including a cane, can work against you because it actually deconditions your muscles. If you need an aid, try to use it for as short a time as possible so you will start using your muscles again.

If walking is difficult for you because your legs are weak; your balance is not as good as it used to be and you may fall; your knees are painful; it's too hot, too cold, or even icy out; or the air quality is poor, there are aerobic exercises you can do at home. Riding a stationary bike is a good one. Stationary bicycles and elliptical trainers are nonimpact machines, which means there's no pounding on the ankles, knees, hip joints, or spine.

You can keep track of your heart rate by wearing a heart rate monitor. Some exercise machines have built-in heart rate monitors. You can also use the old-fashioned, low-tech method of taking your pulse. Your target heart rate for aerobic exercise should be set by your doctor or an exercise specialist who communicates with your doctor, and your rate will relate to your medical condition and the shape you're in. Biking requires a lot of lower extremity strength, especially in the quadriceps. As you exercise targeted muscles, the heart sends blood and therefore oxygen to that muscle group. Aerobic exercise also decreases your resting heart rate and your blood pressure. Exercising your heart challenges it, which helps it do a lot better when it's not challenged.

Resistance Exercises

These exercises challenge targeted muscles through a certain number of repetitions. Usually you will start with one set of repetitions, then in future sessions go to two sets with a brief rest in between the two. Examples of resistance exercises are knee extensions and hamstring curls done with weights strapped to your ankles or sitting on a machine such as a home gym; lifting your hips off a training table or a mat on the floor while squeezing a ball between your knees and again with a ball under your legs; or lying down and opening and closing your knees with an elastic theraband around your thighs for resistance. Rotating the trunk of your body and doing rowing exercises with resistance therabands are other examples of resistance exercises. Squats and lunges are practical exercises that help prepare your body to get out of a chair or up off the floor.

If you use a machine such as a leg press, the resistance comes from the weights stacked on the leg press as, sitting down or lying on your back, you push a heavy bar down with your feet, until your knees are almost straightened out, and then bring your knees back up. The amount of resistance is easy to control because you can add weights to the machine or take them off, making the pushing exercise more difficult or easier. Typically, you don't have to physically lift weights onto the machine and take them back off. The machine is made with a column of weights, and you simply insert a metal pin into the weight level that is correct for you.

To determine the appropriate weight a person should use in doing an exercise, the AHA Science Advisory Committee says to first find out the maximum amount of weight the individual can push when doing that exercise. Then take only a percentage of that maximum. Starting out, that would be 30 percent to 40 percent for the upper body and 50 percent to 60 percent for the hips and legs. "Most studies of previously sedentary adults with and without heart disease, including those with heart failure, reported training workloads of 50 percent to 80 percent" of maximum weight the person could tolerate, the advisory committee reported. If you or your trainer or therapist has any doubts about your ability to test your maximum weight-bearing strength for an exercise, don't do it and just approximate it based on what weight you comfortably handle, the committee advises. Dr. Stewart adds. "For most people, if they can lift a weight 12 to 15 times before having to stop, that weight corresponds to about 50 percent of their maximum capacity."

It is very important for people with a heart problem to use the *correct breathing pattern* while doing resistance exercises. To avoid putting strain on your heart, exhale on the part of the exercise that takes exertion, and inhale on the part that does not, as you return to your normal position.

Times to exhale:

- when you push the leg press down with your feet
- when you push up from a squat
- as you do an ab crunch
- as you move your legs up in a leg curl
- as you curl your arm upward in a bicep curl

By using this breathing pattern, Randy instructs, you don't build pressure. He explains: "That's one of the biggest concerns with people with heart trouble—that they'll get on a machine, and they'll try to do a certain amount of weight, and they'll hold their breath, and everything builds up inside. Their blood pressure increases, and that's where they

---

Recommendations for the Initial Prescription of Resistance Training

Resistance training should be performed

- **in a rhythmical manner at a moderate-to-slow controlled speed;**
- **through a full range of motion, avoiding breath holding and straining (Valsalva maneuver), by exhaling during the contraction or exertion phase of the lift and inhaling during the relaxation phase; and**
- **alternating between upper and lower body work, to allow for adequate rest between exercises.**

The initial resistance or weight load should

- **allow for, and be limited to, 8 to 12 repetitions/set for healthy sedentary adults, or 10 to 15 repetitions at a low level of resistance, for example, ≤ 40% of 1 repetition maximum for older (> 50–60 years of age), more frail persons, and for cardiac patients;**
- **be limited to a single set, performed 2 days per week; and**
- **involve the major muscle groups of the upper and lower extremities, for example, chest press, shoulder press, triceps extension, biceps curl, pull-down (upper back), lower back extension, abdominal crunch/curl-up, quadriceps extension or leg press, leg curls (hamstrings), and calf raise.**

Source: **American Heart Association Science Advisory, *Resistance Exercise in Individuals with and without Cardiovascular Disease: 2007 Update.***

get into a lot of trouble, and that's why people with heart conditions may think that exercise is bad."

Breathing correctly while doing strength training is not automatic with me. I have to think about my breathing and remember when to exhale and when to inhale. I know this is the case because Randy continually prompts me to exhale when I'm exerting myself. At least I'm not aware of holding my breath. Never hold your breath deliberately when straining. But it may happen briefly. "Some breath-holding is unavoidable," Dr. Stewart says, "but try to avoid extended holding and strain. Too much strain can raise the blood pressure to very high levels, which puts unnecessary strain on the heart."

Balance Exercises

Exercises such as standing on a balance board or wobble board are important because balance plays a role in stability and strength. If you don't have good balance, something needs to assist you. You're going to focus more and use muscles a lot harder than a person who has good balance, or you will hold on to something such as a cane, a crutch, or a walker to take the stress off. Randy says that, unless you have an injury, if you use a walking aid, what you are doing is making up for your lack of balance and strength.

YOUR ENVIRONMENT AND YOUR ROUTINE

Once you have learned what exercises to do, and you feel confident that you are doing them correctly, you can continue them on your own. You may go to a facility such as a gym, or you may work out at home. You may be able to find a trainer or physical therapist who is an exercise specialist and is willing to stop by your home periodically to supervise your workout. Or you may return once a month to your cardiac rehabilitation or sports therapy program. Checking in with an expert periodically is a big help for several reasons:

- Knowing that an expert will be watching you who can tell if you are in the shape you should be in will help to keep you honest, exercising regularly.
- Your trainer or therapist can see that you are doing all your exercises correctly, to avoid injury and get the most benefit.

- This expert in body conditioning can tell if it's time for you to move on to a higher level of intensity in some of your exercises or if it's time to introduce a new exercise.

When I decided to take exercising seriously, I turned a room at home into a gym. Everything in the room is devoted to exercising: At first I got an exercise bike for my aerobic exercise; a training table, elastic therabands, ankle weights, and various size exercise balls for doing stretching and resistance exercises; and a stepping board and balance board. But then after several months, I found I wanted more. I needed to strengthen my leg and arm muscles and the core of my body. The ankle weights I used to do leg extensions and leg curls were too easy for me. So I bought a home gym with a leg press.

Whoa! you might say. That's more than I want to do and more than I want to spend. And you don't have to. Not everyone has to do exactly the same thing. If you are able to walk for 20 to 30 minutes every day outdoors or in a shopping mall or wherever you find a convenient place, you can accomplish your exercise without any major piece of equipment. I don't, however, recommend walking around and around in your house or apartment. I tried that, and you can get a pace going and not notice where you're putting your foot and stumble over a toy or a cat or a dog or a lamp cord or whatever may be in your path, not to mention you can start to get dizzy because you're walking in circles through various rooms. And 20 to 30 minutes is a long time to walk in circles. Either walk outdoors or in a covered mall or other large area, or indoors on a treadmill that has handlebars you can hold onto on both sides.

If you do walk as your main aerobic heart-strengthening exercise, you will still need some exercise aids at home—either a floor mat or training table and resistance therabands and balls and weights for resistance training.

KEEPING ON KEEPING ON

My incentive to exercise is strong, yet I found it hard to keep up all my exercise on my own. Monday, Wednesday, and Friday, I do an hour-long exercise routine that combines stretching, aerobic, and resistance exercises. Tuesday, Thursday, and Saturday, I do a shorter routine that leaves out the resistance exercises because muscles need to rest a day from that type of exercise. Six days a week I ride the bike. I started with 5 minutes and went to 10 minutes, then 20 minutes. My future goal is 30 minutes a day. I'm not there yet but would like to be. If 20 or 30 minutes is too long to stay on the bicycle at one sitting, break up your cycling and do half in the morning and half in the afternoon or evening.

To stick to this much exercise day after day, I truly need some help from friends. I am so very fortunate to have my trainer, Randy, who supervises me regularly at home. He left me a daily exercise grid, where I write down how long I work out on the bike, and a checklist of strengthening and stretching exercises to complete daily or every other day. I also write down comments if a part of me hurts, if I feel like I pulled something, or if I found that on this day I did an exercise much easier than before. If I do well, Randy increases the level of exercises the next week: he makes them harder so that I get more benefit from them. There's a limit on how hard he makes them, of course. In a person who has or has had a heart problem, you never want to have so much weight or so many repetitions that you strain to lift the weight.

You may not have a trainer working with you once a week, but you could ask a family member or friend to join you at workouts. Minutes on the bike or treadmill seem to pass much more quickly when you're having a conversation. If you do exercise alone, as you pedal you might want to watch a sports event or other television program or a movie, listen to music, or read a book or magazine article. Book holders are available that slip over the front of a stationary bike.

For those days in between my trainer's visits, I found I still needed help. So I pumped up my environment. I ordered posters and photos of my favorite athletes and put them up on all the walls of my exercise room. Women's soccer titan Mia Hamm keeps me disciplined; iron men Cal Ripken, Jr., and Lou Gehrig make me not want to miss a day; quarterbacks Brady Quinn and Tom Brady show me what body conditioning can lead to. Derek Jeter is my captain; Brett Favre is my inspiration. These guys and other athletes cheer me on in "our" workout room, where on one wall hangs a replica of the Notre Dame sign those football players touch before running out onto the field: "Play like a champion today." Let's do whatever it takes to keep our body power in pace with our mind and soul power.

14

The Patient-Doctor Therapeutic Relationship

> The good physician knows his patients through and through, and his knowledge is bought dearly. Time, sympathy and understanding must be lavishly dispensed, but the reward is to be found in that personal bond, which forms the greatest satisfaction of the practice of medicine. One of the essential qualities of the clinician is interest in humanity, for the secret of the caring of the patient is in the caring for the patient.
>
> —Francis Weld Peabody, M.D. (1881–1927)

The exemplary Harvard physician and teacher, Dr. Peabody, spoke a simple and timeless truth in his classic essay "The Care of the Patient." The doctor you choose to look after your heart is someone you will likely know for a long time, maybe for the rest of your life. Find someone you trust and can talk easily with, someone who answers all your questions and explains as much as you want to know about your situation and the diagnostic tests and treatments you are advised to take. You may find this trust in the very first doctor you see. Or you may have to keep looking. In my journey with heart failure, the first experiences I (Mary) had with doctors made me realize what I didn't have.

When my first cardiologist told me I had heart failure in January 2003, I was shocked. I'm sure I was like you in wanting to ask my doctor lots of questions, find out what had happened, and then develop the best treatment plan. As I mention in the introduction to this book, my first three cardiologists did not put me on the medications that, I found through my own research, were recommended for heart failure treatment in guidelines issued jointly by the American College of Cardiology and the American Heart Association. I continued to do very poorly.

Beyond this significant matter of whether I was getting the most effective treatment, other issues prevented the bond of trust Dr. Peabody calls for. I needed to talk to my first cardiologist about a new medication he put me on, but his staff said he did not accept phone calls from patients; the second cardiologist, who gave me an angiogram, did not tell me immediately afterward or ever that I had died on the table during the procedure and had to be resuscitated (a technician present told me, and I saw the burn marks on my chest from the electric paddles), yet the doctor refused to see me when I was hospitalized after the event; the third cardiologist urged me repeatedly to go on a heart transplant waiting list even though I was not yet prescribed either an ACE inhibitor or a beta blocker, two basic medicines I found recommended for heart failure in the national treatment guidelines. I said no to a heart transplant and, feeling under much stress, searched for yet another cardiologist. This time I found one who knew what to do for me, and I still have my good old biological heart, which improved to normal. I no longer have heart failure.

So first of all, what I want in a doctor is someone who keeps up with the medical literature and national treatment guidelines and will give me the most effective and life-prolonging treatments. I want a doctor to know the scientific basis for the treatments she prescribes. Treatment based on scientific research proving it works is called *evidence-based medicine*—medicine based on evidence that it helps people with a certain illness get better and, in some cases, extends lives. If a doctor recommends treating me with medications that do not have proof that they work, I want to be told that this is the case, and I want to discuss with my doctor whether and why I should take these medications.

I want a doctor to be there for me. I want to feel secure that if something goes wrong, he will really care and try to help. Your doctor can ease your stress, just by letting you know he recognizes what's wrong and knows what to do to help. I want to be able to reach my doctor by phone or e-mail occasionally if I have a question that I believe is important. I want us to have mutual respect and consideration for one another. The best doctor-patient relationships are formed, as Dr. Peabody suggests, through an investment of time spent getting to know one another and building a bond of trust. This relationship begins with the office visit. A patient should come on time, prepared with questions and medical history written down. A doctor understandably may get stacked up with patients, and may need to work on an unscheduled emergency case. Those of us left in the waiting room need to set our patience meter for the duration and read a magazine or book. But it is not okay in general for a patient to sit in the waiting room or an exam room for 30 minutes beyond her appointment time, while the doctor expects all patients to come 5 to 15 minutes early. This patient-doctor encounter should be based on mutual respect for one another as people and for one another's time.

My doctor has to be truthful. If something goes wrong during my treatment, I want to be told about it. I know that, like all of us, doctors sometimes make mistakes, and sometimes things go wrong when the doctor is not at fault. But a patient has a right to know what happens to her, and her doctor has an obligation to tell the truth.

A person with heart failure must commit beyond the doctor's office to personal responsibility for her daily health, taking prescribed medicines, eating a healthy diet, exercising, and becoming fully engaged in life if her health improves. In today's expensive world of medical care, with the heavy influence of pharmaceutical and device companies, high-cost technology, and a health insurance reimbursement system that favors doing procedures over preventive care, you the consumer need, more than ever, to do your homework and get involved in deciding with your doctor what care is best for you.

You want your doctor to get to know you. Caring works both ways. Get to know your doctor, too. You may not have thought much about doctor-patient relationships or how to get the most out of your office visit with your doctor. In the rest of this chapter, Ed Kasper shares the wisdom of his many years of experience caring for people with heart failure. When we named this chapter, Ed inserted the word "therapeutic." I thought I understood what he meant, but asked him to talk about it. He does that beautifully in the next part of the chapter.

Mary Knudson

FORMING A THERAPEUTIC RELATIONSHIP

When doctors speak of a "therapeutic" relationship, what they mean is that something about the relationship actually improves the health of the patient. It is more than the prescriptions given or the procedures performed. There is something here that goes beyond all that. The foundation is caring. Knowing that you are not alone on this trail because you will be guided by a competent, caring doctor is therapeutic. People feel better knowing this.

Wearing my scientist's hat, I suspect that the benefit of the relationship has much to do with stress reduction. Stress is a part of medical illness—the unknown, the painful, the life threatening. In chapter 1 we describe stress and heart failure occurring with an outpouring of hormones such as norepinephrine and angiotensin II, which are beneficial in the short run but detrimental in the long run. We use beta blockers and angiotensin-converting enzyme inhibitors to counteract this hormonal stimulation. We can also reduce stress with a kind word, a caring touch, a knowing smile. While I cannot prove it with a double-blind, randomized, controlled clinical trial, I bet that stress reduction is good for all of us and is a critical component of the truly therapeutic relationship.

How do we form a genuine therapeutic relationship? A great part of this is based on trust. Do you trust me? If you do not, move on to another cardiologist. Most physicians do not mind, and in fact will absolutely support, a second opinion; but if you find yourself constantly questioning every suggestion I make, there must be something wrong. Be knowledgeable, and be informed. Read up on your disease—you are already doing that by reading this book. Good for you. But remember, you pay me for my time, opinion, expertise, and knowledge. I have been living cardiology for a long time, and eventually if you stick with me as your doctor, it should be because you trust that what I say is correct and because we decide together to proceed appropriately. Trust is a cornerstone of this relationship.

The other cornerstone is caring. If you get the sense that I do not care for you as a person or that I am not interested in you as a patient, you should find another cardiologist. Without caring, I am just a technician or a guy capable of doing some interesting procedures. Caring for others has to permeate every fiber of my being. Science is a tool. Caring is why I use this tool. I could not be a research scientist. I enjoy using what I have learned to care for others, and I like to see the results myself. Pure science does not allow me to make that connection. Only medicine allows me to use science for the direct benefit of others.

Honesty must support both trust and caring. I need your honest answers in order to make the proper diagnosis. I will ask you personal questions such as whether you use illicit drugs and whether you drink alcohol. Honest answers help me help you. I will be honest with you in return. There are things you need to know, and I will tell it as I see it, but I will do so in a caring, thoughtful manner.

Telling people good news—that they are getting better—is an easy and enjoyable part of being a doctor. I am asked if it is hard to care for people and yet have to tell them bad news or see them die. Delivering bad news to people you care for is never easy, and I do not like to do it. But if you care for someone, you understand that they need to know the truth so that they can make informed decisions about further medical care, financial issues, legal issues, and personal matters. They may need to say good-bye to an estranged friend or family member. I view the delivery of bad news as part of what it is to be a doctor, but it is never easy. Many nights I awake in the early morning hours worried about how best to tell a patient, someone I now feel is a friend, news I know this person will not want to hear. The delivery of bad news must be done gently, carefully, and thoughtfully. There are tears, and it can be emotionally gut wrenching for all of us—the patient, the family members, the doctor.

I remember telling one patient and his wife that he needed a heart transplant. This was not an easy discussion. That room on Osler 4 in Johns Hopkins Hospital seemed so small, and the patient and his wife looked similar to me and my wife in age. I walked away from that room thinking, "That could be me," all the while admiring this family's strength. Sometimes you get to see the absolute best in people, and this was one of those times. I felt they comforted me more than I comforted them.

Death faces us all. I carry with me in my soul a little bit of everyone for whom I have ever cared. Some of these people have died, some will die shortly, and others may outlive me. As a physician, I have the opportunity and responsibility to heal others. If this is not possible, I still have the responsibility to provide comfort. This often means a frank talk about end-of-life issues. It sometimes means holding the hand of a patient or a family member when nothing more curative can be offered. It may mean pain control, and it may also mean a kind touch, a few extra minutes spent reminiscing, or recognition of this person's importance to family, friends, and me. Being a doctor means providing comfort, conversation, and companionship, even—or especially—when I have nothing else to offer.

I enjoy getting to know my patients. It has been a privilege to meet and care for so many fine people over the past 20-something years. Why don't you get to know your cardiologist a little? Ask me about my son. Find out what I like to do with my spare time. I am probably going to ask you the same. All of this goes toward building the trust and caring that forms the therapeutic relationship. As your cardiologist, I will already know a lot about you. But you should also want me to know your goals and desires as well. Just not all at once and at the first visit! There will be time enough for this relationship to develop, and it does take time, just as any friendship takes time. I should say that joking about malpractice is never appreciated and is not funny. Humor, though, is always appreciated. It makes the day better to see a smile and hear a funny story. Being upbeat is infectious.

Planning Your Office Visit

Your cardiologist is running a small business. I sell my time, caring, and expertise. A typical first-time visit might last an hour, and a return visit might last 20 minutes. I will then need to move on to the next person. To make the most of our time together, you need to prepare.

Assume that you are scheduled for a visit in my office. How do you make the best use of our time together? Be prepared. Be organized. Be succinct, and be friendly. Do some homework beforehand. Know your medical history and perhaps even write it down in chronological order with dates. Give me a copy of this history, or better still, send the history and your medical records in advance and make sure they have been received. I like to review your records the night before I see you for the first time. In this way, I can spend the time we have allotted interacting *with you* and not hunched over your medical records while you sit quietly in the room.

Bring a referral if your insurance requires this, as well as all of your insurance information. Bring a list of your medications or the medications themselves. Bring a list of questions. Finally, bring a list of your physicians' names and addresses. More likely than not, you have been told to see me by another physician. You want to make sure that I send my opinion to all your other doctors so that we will all be on the same page. If you spend some time in preparation, you will spend less time doing paperwork with me and more time focusing on your problem. Preparation and organization are the keys.

You should expect me, and every other cardiologist, to be kind, patient, caring, and knowledgeable. You should expect a sense of decorum and privacy. You should expect that I will follow up if I say I will follow up and will call when I say I will call. You should expect me to be on time. You should be on time as well.

Any small business should value critical feedback. If my office staff did something particularly good or bad, let me know about it. I aim for excellence, and when we hit it right, it is great to hear about it. When we miss, I need to hear about that as well.

You have now finished your appointment and are returning to the real world, armed with a prescription for a drug or a request for a test. Maybe you got some good news and maybe you didn't. The next part is all yours. Take your medications as directed. If you have questions, ask. Show up for the ordered procedures on time and prepared as directed. Keep a diary of symptoms and your daily weight. You will find that a rapid gain in weight will often signal an increase in fluid retention and precede congestion. Watch the salt in your diet and follow your doctor's nutritional and exercise recommendations (see chapters 12 and 13). Don't smoke. Learn as much as you can about heart failure and what caused the heart failure in you. Know your ejection fraction. To summarize, here is how a patient can help me in the therapeutic relationship.

How Patients Can Help Me to Help Them

- Pay attention. It is only natural to zone out, but if I am not making myself clear, ask questions. It is your health after all.
- Be active. Participate in your health care. I cannot improve your health all by myself, and neither can you. It takes both of us to get you better.
- Be honest and open. I cannot help if I do not know what really happened. Do you think I have never before heard anything like the story you are going to tell me? Think again.
- Take responsibility. Not everything in life is under our control, but you can be responsible for things that are, like your diet, taking your medications, and exercise.

- Be friendly. Like most things in life, you will get better service if you ask with a smile rather than a frown.
- Be patient. Not everything will always go smoothly. I will sometimes be late. Lab data might get lost temporarily. Things happen. Try to go with the flow. Do not be shy, however, if something is really wrong.
- Get organized. I have said it before and will say it again: the organized patient simply does better. Disorganization leads to mistakes. This is especially true when dealing with multiple medications. Develop as close to a foolproof way as you can to keep your medications organized. Many people use a pill sorter and set out their week's medications in advance. This kind of organization decreases mistakes.
- Respect timeliness. Be on time yourself, and try to be aware of other people's time. Be succinct. Long rambling answers to yes or no questions are unhelpful.
- Prepare. Much like the good Boy Scout, prepare for visits to your doctor. Bring your medication list, and don't leave it in your vehicle. Send records in advance so that they can be reviewed before your visit.
- Laugh when you can. Humor is often the best medicine. It certainly makes for a more cheerful and upbeat day.
- Be aware. Be aware of changes in your medical condition. Call me with the first signs of deterioration. Don't wait until you have to be hospitalized.

TIPS FOR LIVING WELL WITH HEART FAILURE

When you travel, take enough medications with you in your travel bag for the entire trip—plus some, just in case. Keep another full set in your checked baggage in case you lose your travel bag. Keep an outline of your medical history with you. That way, if you need to see a local doctor while you are away from home, she will not be starting from scratch.

Keep an eye on your symptoms. Are you getting short of breath with less and less exertion? Do you find yourself waking up at night short of breath? Do you feel your heart racing or skipping beats? Do you feel lightheaded? Have you fainted? Do you have more chest pain? All of these are reasons to consult your doctor. In fact, any change in your symptoms for the worse is a good reason to speak with your doctor.

Be prepared to deal with problems. Do you know where the hospital emergency room is? If you call an ambulance to your house for an emergency, the paramedics typically have orders to take you to the hospital emergency room closest to your house. That may not be the hospital where your doctor practices, but you may need to go there because it is the closest. Know how to get to that hospital and where to park. Your family may need to drive you there, you never know. If you do have a choice in hospitals, ask your cardiologist which one he recommends.

Speak with your physician. Tell me about your symptoms and the results of treatment. It is better to catch a potential problem early than to wait until you need to be hospitalized. The worsening of symptoms tends to occur rapidly, more rapidly than you would predict based on experience. Do not assume that "it can wait until I see my doctor next week." You may end up seeing me tonight in the emergency room.

Listen to your doctor. If I say you need to go to the hospital, get there quickly. I do not take hospitalization lightly. If I say you need to be hospitalized, it is either because I cannot effectively treat you as an outpatient or because it would be dangerous to do so.

Realize that your goals may change over time. You may start out thinking that quantity of life is more important than quality of life. With the passage of time, you may get to the point where quality of life is paramount. This is not giving up; this is simply a change in priorities. Let me know about your priorities. Make sure your physicians and family know your wishes regarding end-of-life care. You may not be able to express your wishes when you are really ill. Now is the time to make them known. A living will is a good way to document your wishes for whether and under what circumstances you would want such life-prolonging measures as being placed on an artificial respirator that breathes for you or having a feeding tube in your stomach if you are unable to eat. I encourage you to complete this document. You can obtain a blank form from your health department, from your lawyer, or through the Internet. Nothing, however, takes the place of an honest discussion with your loved ones and physician.

Miracles happen every day in hospitals and physician offices across the country and around the world. Every year I care for people whose initial ejection fraction is horrible. Yet with the right drugs at the right doses coupled with a healthy dose of caring, many of these people get substantially better. Your knowledge about heart failure and its treatments gives you the best possible chance for a miracle to occur. I hope a miracle of modern medicine occurs for you.

Ed Kasper

Getting to Know Your Doctor

Who is your doctor? If she is anything like me, she was probably the kid in high school who really liked science. I enjoy knowing how things work. Like me, your doctor probably did very well in school. This is not enough, however, to be a good doctor. I made the decision to become a physician rather than a scientist because I like helping people, and I enjoy using science to benefit individuals. If I did not enjoy the immediate gratification of helping people deal with illness, I would have become something else.

To understand your cardiologist, I think it helps to know a little about his training. I knew from seventh grade on that I wanted to be a physician. Miss Pasteur taught seventh-grade human biology in the Wilton, Connecticut, Middle School. She inspired in me a desire to know more about how we work. I completed four years of college at Johns Hopkins University in Baltimore, Maryland, majoring in natural sciences, which meant taking many more science classes. I then spent another four years at the University of Connecticut School of Medicine in Farmington, Connecticut. (These days, I would be in the minority, as the typical medical school class is more than 50 percent female.)

In medical school, I spent the first two years in the classroom learning about normal and abnormal human structure and function. In the third and fourth years, I moved to the hospital and outpatient clinic, where I began to learn what taking care of patients really means and how this is done. I saw my first patient in the second week of medical school. During the first two years, we learned to take patient histories and do physical examinations by going to the hospital to see patients one afternoon a week. That first visit was just a chance to speak with a patient, the first time I smelled that hospital smell. I walked into the room and sat down, feeling insignificant and hopelessly inept. The patient was hospitalized with bowel obstruction and had a tube passed through his nose and into his stomach to drain it. Contents of his stomach collected in a bottle on the floor. I shyly asked him if that tube hurt, and his response was "What do you think?" I was green and naïve, and, frankly, it looked like it really hurt.

During my next year as an intern at Johns Hopkins Hospital, I basically lived in the hospital. If medical school is like learning French in a classroom, internship is like being dropped in Paris with $50 and told to figure out how to live there for a year. My first day of internship was a Sunday. I admitted only one patient, a woman who was very sick, and I wondered if I was good enough and smart enough to be in that room at all, much less taking care of her with the help of others more senior than I. Two weeks later, she left the hospital, and I was on top of the world.

Internship was followed by two years of residency, also at Johns Hopkins Hospital, where I completed the process of training in internal medicine and learned how to supervise interns. At the end of residency and passing a certifying examination, I was a board-certified internist. I spent a year as one of four chief residents in the Internal Medicine Department at Hopkins. To this day, the chief residents are called assistant chiefs of service. I supervised a team of thirty interns and residents as we provided care to patients admitted to a thirty-bed unit called Osler 4, named after the first chief of medicine at Johns Hopkins Hospital, Sir William Osler. These were the most exciting years of my life. I was young, doing something that really mattered, and the learning curve was steep. Every day I learned something new.

This was followed by three years of cardiology fellowship at Johns Hopkins Hospital. During fellowship, I learned to be a cardiologist. My first cardiac catheterization was a daunting experience. I might have gotten four hours of sleep the night before as I studied how to do the procedure. It went flawlessly, and I finally felt like a cardiologist. I did additional training in heart failure and heart transplantation but could just as easily have chosen electrophysiology, echocardiography, or interventional cardiology. I chose this field because the patients interested me, and I thought I could make a difference. At that time, 1989, you could have a meeting of all the cardiologists interested in caring for heart transplant recipients gathered around a large table. I was getting into something important at the beginning, and that was very attractive. After fellowship and passing another certifying examination, I became board certified in cardiovascular diseases. To maintain these certifications, a doctor must pass examinations and meet other requirements every 10 years.

From college, it is not unusual to spend 12 or more years in training to become a cardiologist and even more to become a cardiac surgeon. During my training, the hours were long, and the pay was short. I was on call every third night, usually sleeping in the hospital. Educational loans became due, and money was tight. I was very lucky. I had excellent mentors all along the way, beginning with Miss Pasteur and continuing up to the people I work with this very day. I received nothing but thoughtful training at several outstanding institutions. I look back on this training with respect for those who cared enough to care about me and gratitude for the friends I made along the way.

Most cardiologists are in practice with one or more others. The average cardiology group has about five cardiologists. I work with over eighty at the Johns Hopkins Medical Institutions. Some days are spent mostly seeing outpatients; others mostly caring for patients in the hospital. To these clinical responsibilities, academic cardiologists (those like me who are in practice at a medical school) also add teaching responsibilities and research. Days can be very busy, nights can be very long, and your cardiologist is likely being pulled in several different directions. While you will have a primary cardiologist you get to know well, don't be surprised if occasionally you have to see another doctor who works in the same office. In general, the practice assumes responsibility for your care when your cardiologist is unavailable. With the aging of our population and the increase in demand for cardiovascular services, an obvious problem looms on the horizon. There will be too many patients for too few cardiologists.

Getting to know your cardiologist makes good sense. It helps to develop the therapeutic relationship. Understanding how your cardiologist got to where he is today may help you make that connection.

E. K.

15

What You Need to Know about the Hospital

The most frequent cause for a trip to the hospital in people age 65 or older is heart failure. A hospital is a place where people come to get help, and many, many of them do. Unfortunately, some people are also harmed in the hospital. In this chapter, we discuss what brings heart failure patients to the hospital, what you can expect in hospital care, and what you can do to make your hospital stay safer.

WHY DO PEOPLE WITH HEART FAILURE NEED HOSPITALIZATION?

Most people with heart failure will be hospitalized at some point in the course of their illness. Usually the reason is too much fluid accumulated in the body that is making it hard to breathe and causing the heart to labor. People who are so fatigued that it is difficult for them to get out of bed often benefit from a brief stay in the hospital to remove their excess fluid. If, in addition to fluid accumulation, fatigue, and shortness of breath, the person has low blood pressure and kidney problems, he is in real trouble. Such signs suggest that the heart is no longer capable of generating an adequate blood pressure to provide blood flow that will allow the kidneys to do their job properly. This is one of the ways in which people with severe heart failure die.

Different reasons bring people with heart failure to a hospital. They may be hospitalized when they are first diagnosed with heart failure. Or they know they have heart failure but didn't watch the salt in their diet, were taking inadequate medications, or were unable or unwilling to take their medications, and consequently got too much fluid buildup. Sometimes, an environment is too hot, too cold, or too stressful. Sometimes, their hospitalization is simply due to the progression of their disease. Whatever the reason, at some point many people exceed what doctors can do to treat them as an outpatient, and they need the benefits of a hospital stay.

The short amount of time it takes to reach an emergency condition may catch you by surprise.

> *One of my patients first came to see me (Ed) with atrial flutter and a fast heart rate. He was 60 years old, didn't have heart failure, and had no history of heart attack. I made some changes in his medications and spoke with his doctor about his treatment. He lives far from Baltimore, where he had traveled to see me. He went home and missed several appointments with me but finally came back to see me one day three months later. He was very sick. He had gained almost 30 pounds, and all of it was fluid. His ankles and legs were massive and filled with fluid. He could no longer wear shoes and instead wore house slippers. His waist had markedly increased in size. He had to wear sweatpants because they could expand to fit him. He had difficulty breathing at rest and couldn't lie down without getting markedly short of breath. He was trying to sleep in a chair, and even in this position, he woke up many times at night gasping for air.*
>
> *He had failed to take his medications and was so depressed that he didn't return to his doctors. By the time he did, he had many of the typical symptoms of heart failure brought on by dilated cardiomyopathy, including such severe shortness of breath that even simple things such as dressing had become major undertakings. I admitted him to the hospital right away.*

Dr. Sheldon Gottlieb, a cardiologist at the Johns Hopkins Bayview Medical Center, points out that we humans have a tendency to think in straight lines—this is termed linear thinking. We simply do not think in curves—so-called nonlinear thinking. Instead, we think, I am feeling bad today, but I have an appointment with my doctor on Monday—three days from now. We extrapolate from past experience that if we feel bad today, then by Monday, if we continue to worsen in a straight line, we will be only so much worse. We don't realize that the worsening of heart failure symptoms right before a hospitalization is not a straight line but occurs much more rapidly, in a nonlinear manner. Because of this, we end up in the emergency room on Sunday night. Dr. Gottlieb calls this the "nonlinear patient trap," and I have seen it happen again and again. An early call to your doctor may help prevent an admission to the hospital, or at least an emergency admission.

If you have a choice, you would rather come through the hospital admitting office than the emergency room. Sometimes you may be so sick that you simply need to call 911 and go by ambulance to the nearest ER. Other times, your doctor may be able to arrange for you to be admitted, bypassing the ER experience. When you truly need the emergency room, it is a miraculous place. If you are not extremely ill, however, the ER will likely mean a long wait to be seen, uncomfortable surroundings, and people you have never met before. If you are well enough to do so, avoid this experience. Call and visit your doctor when you first suspect you have a problem. Do not delay.

HOSPITAL THERAPY FOR EXCESS FLUID

Since the major reason for hospitalizing a patient with heart failure is accumulation of fluid, the primary goal of therapy is very simple: remove the excess water. Accomplishing this simple goal, however, can have dangerous side effects, and patients must be carefully monitored. The major medications to do this are intravenous: loop diuretics dripped directly into a vein. *Loop diuretic* means the diuretic works in the kidney on the loop of Henle, the part where much of the sodium and water is reabsorbed. Intravenous loop diuretics work better than those taken orally simply because more of the drug is absorbed and travels to the kidneys, causing increased urination. In severe heart failure, not only the feet and ankles, but the gut and liver are swollen with fluid as well. This excess fluid in the gut and liver decreases absorption of medications swallowed, and that is why diuretic pills a person takes at home may not give enough relief. Giving the same medications by vein works better. This is especially true of the loop diuretics. Typically, an intravenous loop diuretic will be given between one and three times a day and should result in a brisk need to urinate. If a patient can't use a bathroom, a catheter is often inserted, but it is removed as quickly as possible to try to prevent infection.

Most patients who need to be hospitalized to get rid of excess fluid are not sick enough to go to the coronary care unit, where people get more intensive care, and will go onto a hospital floor. The typical hospital room still contains two beds; one for you, and one for your new roommate. Most of us have not shared a room with anyone other than our spouse in decades. This lack of privacy remains a major source of frustration. The hospital of the future will contain only single-bed rooms, but right now this is not the case. Many hospitals have "high amenities" floors, which contain single-bed rooms and the atmosphere of a luxury hotel. If you can afford the extra charge, not covered by your insurance, such a floor may be the way to go. Privacy is important because you will be discussing very personal issues, and it is nice to do so separated by more than a curtain.

During diuretic treatment, we measure *I's and O's,* which is simply your fluid input and output. My patient with 30 pounds of fluid quickly started losing it. His output was more than his input by about 1.5 liters a day. This resulted in a nice decrease in his body weight, also measured daily. He began to feel better within three days, and within a week had lost enough fluid to be able to sleep in a bed once again.

If intravenous loop diuretics are not as effective as desired, the dose can be increased or combined with an intravenous thiazide diuretic to cause more fluid loss. But this must be done with caution and vigilance. Higher doses and a combination of a loop diuretic and a thiazide diuretic lead to more side effects and complications, such as low blood potassium and magnesium that must be replaced. High-dose loop diuretics and combinations of diuretics must be carefully adjusted to achieve fluid loss without harming the kidneys.

If this therapy does not cause a brisk loss of fluids, additional intravenous drugs may be used. There are several drugs that quickly decrease the pressure within the heart and lungs. They work by increasing the size of the arteries and veins. Think of a garden hose. If we want to decrease the pressure inside the hose, one way we can do so is by increasing the diameter. Likewise, if we want to increase the pressure inside a hose, we could decrease the diameter. Several different types of drugs increase the diameter of blood vessels. The most commonly used is nitroglycerin. This is the same drug that, when taken under the tongue, is used to treat angina due to a decrease in blood flow in the coronary arteries. It very effectively increases the diameter of veins and arteries and lowers pressure inside the lungs. It is the high pressure within the lungs that leads to wet lungs and shortness of breath. The downside to nitroglycerin is that people become tolerant to its effects when they use it continuously, and it takes a bigger and bigger dose to get the same effect. Another side effect is a splitting headache. So in patients extremely short of breath due to fluid retention, nitroglycerin is often used only temporarily until the loop diuretics start to work.

A close relative of nitroglycerin is nitroprusside, which is given intravenously. This medication is less commonly used because it breaks down when exposed to light and may cause a big drop in blood pressure. It does not cause tolerance as nitroglycerin does.

Nesiritide also lowers pressures inside the heart and lungs. It is the synthetic hormone BNP, or brain natriuretic peptide (see chapter 4). This drug, while very effective, has become controversial. Several studies have documented the effectiveness of nesiritide, but a couple suggest that it leads to more kidney problems than expected and may even decrease survival. A large clinical trial looking at just these issues is under way. If diuretics are not getting the job done, one of these agents—nitroglycerin, nitroprusside, or nesiritide—is combined with a loop diuretic to cause fluid loss and improve symptoms. You may want to discuss with your doctor which one will be used.

THE HOSPITAL STAFF

You will meet many new people in the hospital: nurses, technicians, doctors, nurse's aides, orderlies, social workers, case managers, dietitians, physical therapists, occupational therapists, volunteers, perhaps medical students, interns, and residents, and the list goes on. All are there to help you, although you may wonder if being awakened for a 4 a.m. blood draw could really be termed "help."

The team is led by the attending physician. This person is usually your cardiologist or one of her partners. The attending physician may change with some regularity as partners rotate hospital duties. This is because your doctor will continue to have people to see in the office as well and will work out an arrangement for someone else to see his hospitalized patients. A relatively new development is the hospitalist. This is a doctor who cares only for hospitalized patients and does not see office patients. Insurance companies like hospitalists because by spending all day in the hospital, they move patients more quickly through the system. The downside is that your cardiologist or internist will not have as clear a picture of what happened to you in the hospital if she was not involved directly.

Your nurses will work in 8- or 12-hour shifts. If you are on a regular floor of thirty patients, there may be only two nurses and some technicians to care for all those patients. The role of nurses has changed dramatically in the past twenty years. Not only are they in charge of your comfort, they now also have to be expert in managing a host of bedside technologies, from something as simple as blood sugar testing to something as complicated as a left ventricular assist device. They are the rock on which hospital care is based.

Interns, residents, and fellows have all graduated from medical school and are in various stages of training. The intern is in his first year after graduation. The resident is in her second or third years after graduation. The residents are in charge of the interns. Interns and residents on a medical floor are training to be internists or specialists in internal medicine. Fellows are certified in internal medicine and are now spending three or more years training to become cardiologists. In the middle of the night, an intern, resident, or fellow will most likely be summoned by the nurse to your bedside if something bad happens. Not all hospitals will have interns, residents, or fellows. In those hospitals, hospitalists usually care for the patients during the night.

HOSPITALIZATION FOR LOW BLOOD PRESSURE AND KIDNEY PROBLEMS

The combination of severe heart failure symptoms, low blood pressure (less than 80 mmHg systolic), and kidney problems indicates real trouble. Slightly low blood pressure is healthy, but when the top number in the normal blood pressure reading of 120/80 drops to 80 or below, medical intervention is needed. It suggests that the heart is so weak that it cannot provide enough power to maintain blood pressure and provide adequate blood flow to the kidneys. A person in this condition may need a left ventricular assist device or heart transplantation. In the meantime, one of several drugs may be used to raise blood pressure and improve blood flow to the kidneys. Almost all of these drugs act like the human hormone norepinephrine, which is elevated in heart failure. Intravenous norepinephrine, dopamine, dobutamine, and milrinone will all, to some degree, raise blood pressure by decreasing the diameter of blood vessels, increasing the strength of heart contractions, and increasing heart rate.

If doctors can increase both the amount of blood the heart pumps out with each beat and the heart rate, then blood flow is increased as well. This comes at a cost, however. All drugs used to speed blood flow have been shown to increase death rate when used for more than a week or so in patients with heart failure. There are times, however, when such drugs must be used for a couple of days to get past an immediate problem such as critically low blood pressure. The use of these drugs in such situations is justified in the hopes that the immediate problem can be corrected and the drug stopped quickly.

One young man was confined to a hospital bed and couldn't breathe. He was in true heart failure, his blood pressure was dangerously low, and he was not responding well to standard intravenous diuretics. He was already on dopamine, and despite this he couldn't move without being short of breath. His kidney function was deteriorating rapidly, and the medical team didn't have much time. I discussed the patient with my surgical colleague and the rest of the heart transplant team at our weekly clinical meeting. We decided to give the patient a left ventricular assist device and place him on the heart transplant waiting list. The patient did well with the assist surgery and stayed in the hospital on the assist device until he received a new heart about six months later. He is still doing well today, thanks to modern technology.

People as sick as this young man was are likely to spend time in a hospital's coronary care unit.

THE CORONARY CARE UNIT

A coronary care unit typically has ten to twenty individual rooms, some for critical care and some for intermediate care, facing a nursing station. The patient is attached to an IV and a heart monitor that nurses can track at their desk to see if any major change occurs in heart rate or rhythm or blood pressure. Oxygen is delivered through nasal prongs placed in the nose. A variety of emergency equipment in beige or gray plastic and metal surrounds the head of the bed. As in regular hospital rooms, the patient has a phone and a TV. However, in contrast to hospital floors, in a CCU there will be one nurse for every one to two patients, and that nurse will be more frequently in the room, at least every hour. If a patient is very ill, the nurse may spend most of her shift in the patient's room. A doctor usually visits once to twice a day. Family members are allowed to visit, but not usually around the clock except in special circumstances.

As a patient, you will see and hear unexpected things in the hospital, and intrusions will keep you awake. Doctors and nurses talk in the hall; things are noisy at night. You may watch as a team performs cardiopulmonary resuscitation on the patient in the next room. I have seen the look in other patients' eyes after the emergency team came running with an electrical shock cart to resuscitate a patient on the unit. The fear is very clear, especially if the patient we tried to resuscitate died.

Life in the CCU is stressful not just for patients, but also for their caregivers. When I am on service as the CCU attending physician, my long hours there are always interesting, but often stressful. I supervise a team of medical students, interns, residents, and fellows as we care for anywhere from ten to twenty people suffering from life-threatening heart disease. I start my day early, often very early, because I like to review what happened to the patients overnight. An early start allows me to think in the quiet hours of the early morning about what I want to do for each patient. I review their charts, look at lab work, review medications, and quickly eyeball each patient prior to rounding with my team. Rounds are the central focus of the morning. Starting at 8 a.m. my team and I visit and examine every patient we care for, usually beginning with the sickest.

After examining a patient, we stand outside the room with the person's charts and a laptop connected to the hospital's computer hub. The interns and residents present their findings and ideas on the patient. I question them until I think we have a plan for that person that all understand. We then move on. I try to complete the entire process within four hours because otherwise we are all pulled in other directions. New patients are being admitted to us from the Emergency Department, problems are occurring with other patients, and unless we move along briskly, we will never get done. At the end of rounds, we look at each echocardiogram and cardiac catheterization done the previous day.

The afternoon is filled with new patients and consultations. I see every new patient admitted to the team, and I am often asked to see other patients in the hospital by their doctors. There are test results to review, and families to speak with. The level of medical understanding demonstrated by families as a group and family members individually varies considerably. Some are very up to date; they understand the disease and ask very good questions. Others do not, and some are frankly hostile. Some families are never present, and others are always there. Some people are alone in this world, and others surrounded by friends and relatives. Sickness often brings out the best in people, but sometimes it does not, and at times it reveals deep character flaws. Speaking with family members is a very important part of my day.

There are also other physicians to contact. Sometimes it is the doctor who sent the patient to me in the first place. Or it may be a doctor who will be doing surgery or a procedure on my patients, and I want to make sure we agree about what is to be done. There are nurses and case managers and social workers, all of whom play important roles, and communication among all of us is key.

We care for really sick people, and with that comes a certain level of stress. Are we doing the right thing? Did we forget something? Did we miss something? Are the medications correct? Did we remember to adjust the dose based on the patient's kidney function? These thoughts run through my head all day and well into the night.

People will die in the CCU. Some are just too old and too worn out to get better from something they would have conquered a year ago. Some decide that they have had enough and just wish us to keep them comfortable. Some struggle to the very end but are overtaken by overwhelming infection, untreatable heart failure, unmanageable heart rhythm problems, or a big heart attack.

We all will die. Some deaths are expected, like the person who has kidney failure and decides to stop dialysis. The expected deaths are sad and difficult but somehow less stressful. The unexpected deaths are another thing entirely. This is a time of incredible stress. Did we do something wrong? What could we have done differently? Consoling family members can be gut wrenching.

I usually go home fairly late feeling like I have accomplished something. Sometimes I do save a life, and that is a great feeling. Sometimes I was unable to save a life, but I did comfort the person and his family until the end. That is an accomplishment as well.

ADDITIONAL MANAGEMENT OF YOUR DISEASE

If you are in the hospital with heart failure, you will probably be asked to stay connected to oxygen by wearing a band around your head that holds in place very short tubing you insert in your nostrils. The tubing is hooked to an oxygen outlet that continually blows oxygen into your nose, thereby increasing the amount of oxygen in your bloodstream. The tubing can be uncomfortable. You may want to ask for lubrication to ease the pressure on your nose.

You will also be asked to save all your urine so that the total amount of fluid entering your body (input) and the total amount you excrete (output) can be measured. We want your output to be greater than your input by a liter or so a day. This will lead to about a kilogram (slightly over two pounds) of weight loss per day. As this excess fluid drains from your body, you will feel relief from shortness of breath and swelling of your abdomen, legs, feet, and ankles. If you limit the amount of fluid you drink, you will get quicker relief. You will be given a low-sodium diet. Remember, where sodium goes, water follows, so the less sodium you consume, the less fluid we will have to remove.

For the first day or so, you may spend most of your time in bed. As you get better, getting up and out of bed becomes important. Physical deconditioning occurs very quickly, and more quickly the older you are. If you spend more than several days in bed, you may need the help of a physical therapist to get back on your feet again because of muscle weakness caused by inactivity. We sometimes put an exercise bike in a patient's room, especially someone who is going to be hospitalized for a long time, such as someone waiting for a heart transplant while using a left ventricular assist device. Staying in shape makes for better recovery after the transplant.

In summary, you help yourself when you

- restrict fluids
- save your urine to be measured by your nurse
- follow a low-sodium diet
- get up and out of bed to avoid deconditioning
- take your medications as directed
- bring new problems to the notice of your nurse and doctor immediately

WHAT TO BEWARE OF IN THE HOSPITAL

In a hospital you can improve very quickly. A number of bad things can happen also. Some are simply an annoyance, such as a roommate who snores or other noise or lights on in your room or shining in from the hall. You and your roommate can agree to keep conversations and television at a low level, and you can try to keep your door closed to shut out noise and light from the corridor. But what you really need to be concerned about, and what we discuss here, are things that can go wrong and are life threatening.

Infection

Hospitals are supposed to be kept very clean, and yet germs abound in them. You are particularly at risk if you have a tube going into any part of your body. Anytime you break the defense barrier of the body with an opening through which tubes are placed—in arteries, veins, your bladder, lungs, stomach, or anywhere else—you become more prone to infection. Tubes are a highway on which the bacteria that cover people all the time, and that you will come in contact with from hospital personnel and equipment, can travel directly into your bloodstream, bladder, or lungs. An estimated 1.7 million infections are associated with hospital health care, and 99,000 deaths occur from these infections each year, according to a 2007 report from the Centers for Disease Control and Prevention (CDC). Of these 1.7 million infections, 32 percent are urinary tract infections, 22 percent are surgical site infections, 15 percent are pneumonia (lung infections), and 14 percent are bloodstream infections.

The use and, frankly, sometimes overuse of antibiotics in the hospital have produced a variety of bacteria that are resistant to many of the standard antibiotics. Such superbacteria are difficult to treat.

To limit your chances of catching one of these, you (or your family, if you are unable) should encourage your health care team to get rid of all tubes as soon as they are no longer needed. Keep an eye on your skin where intravenous lines are inserted, and if the area looks infected or hurts, point this out to your nurse. Do not be shy about asking your nurses and doctors to keep your intravenous lines clean. Hand washing is also of the utmost importance. Your doctors and nurses should be washing their hands between each patient with either soap and water or an alcohol-based gel. This simple act has been shown to decrease the hospital infection rate. If you do not see a doctor or nurse wash her hands before approaching your bedside to examine you or to perform a procedure on you, speak up and ask if she will please wash first.

Unfortunately, my out-of-town patient caught the bacterial infection *Staphylococcus aureus,* and it was resistant to many of the usual antibiotics. MRSA (methicillin-resistant *Staphylococcus aureus*) infection is common in hospitals. My patient was treated with vancomycin, an antibiotic that did work, and the infected intravenous line was removed. However, this infection prolonged his hospital stay by at least a week. He eventually went home and has continued to do well. We finally got him out of atrial flutter and back to a normal rhythm. With this, his heart function improved, and heart failure has not been a problem since.

The use of antibiotics also leads to the development of infectious diarrhea. By killing the good bacteria in your gut, you leave behind certain bad bacteria that are not only resistant to the antibiotics but also very infectious. Limiting the duration of antibiotics to just the amount you need and no more will limit your chance of having this bacteria overgrow and cause harm. Some hospitals have better infection-control policing than others, but even in the most closely monitored hospitals, infections occur every day, and the surest way to avoid them is to keep your stay brief.

Other Types of Harm that Occur in Hospitals

Infection is one type of harm that can be reliably predicted to occur to hospitalized patients. There are other, more unpredictable problems. Step back and take a look at what happens in a hospital. A big hospital might have five hundred or even a thousand patients. Each patient is on anywhere from one to twenty medications. Each medication has to be written by a doctor, read and then dispensed by one of many pharmacists, delivered to the floor by one of many different technicians, and finally given to you by one of hundreds of nurses. Almost none of this process is automated, and medication errors occur. Some of them are, unfortunately, deadly. Medication errors would drop if doctors wrote prescriptions into a computer rather than scribbling them on a patient chart, often in hard-to-read handwriting. Patients take medications many times a day. It is a wonder that more medication mistakes don't occur.

Ask your nurse what medication you are taking and why. If you are not getting the medications you normally take at home, get an explanation. The more involved you and your family are, the less likely mistakes are to occur. In order to become involved, you have to know what you are taking at home, at what dose, and how many times a day.

Blood transfusions are another source of error. A blood transfusion can be life saving, but not if the blood type is incorrect. Certain infections can also be transmitted through blood transfusion, for instance, hepatitis and HIV transmission. The blood supply is carefully screened, and your risk is very low. Just the same, blood transfusion should be avoided if at all possible. However, often there is no alternative.

Another area of concern is the wrong surgery, procedure, or test. All procedures are supposed to be preceded by a "time out." Your doctors and nurses should stop before beginning, to make sure you are getting the right procedure at the right time. Help them by wearing the identification bracelet provided by the hospital. Before you are wheeled out of your room to get a test or procedure, know exactly what it is, who ordered it, and why you are getting it. Once at the procedure room, ask the technician or doctor what you are getting and ask what patient's name they have down for this procedure. Before you are put to sleep in an operating room for a surgery, speak to the surgeon and go over exactly what he plans to do on which part of your body.

Things you can do to avoid harm:

- Know your medications and ask your nurse if you see that you are being given something new or are not getting something you normally take at home or at the hospital.
- Discuss your treatment plan with your attending physician.
- Understand why you are getting every procedure, surgery, and test.
- Keep an eye out for infection. Report any redness, swelling, or fever.
- Don't be shy. Make sure your doctors and nurses wash their hands.

IF YOU ARE HOSPITALIZED FOR A REASON OTHER THAN HEART FAILURE

Although you have heart failure, you may be hospitalized with a broken leg or because you need your gallbladder removed or for any of a hundred other things. Again, make sure you stay on your usual medications unless you get a very clear reason why one or more must be discontinued. At the end of your hospitalization, make sure you reconcile what medicines the doctors want you to take at home. If changes in your medications were made during your hospitalization, understand why, and be sure to find out how to take your new drugs. Update your medication list when you get home. Tell your cardiologist immediately if any of your usual heart medications were changed. If, for whatever reason (usually because of surgery), hospital caregivers have changed the settings of your pacemaker or implantable cardioverter defibrillator, make sure it gets reset to your usual settings.

The hospital is a wondrous place where things are done today that doctors only dreamed about even 10 years ago. Many patients feel better and go home more quickly than ever before. There is, however, harm caused in the hospital. Never go to a hospital unless you have to, and when you enter a hospital, know to be on guard. Appoint a family member or friend to be your patient representative. Be aware of potential sources of mistakes and help your health care team avoid them. We hope you avoid the hospital entirely. If you need to be there, may your stay be short and safe.

16

Heart Failure in Elderly People

Heart failure is common in elderly people, so much so that an estimated 10 percent of people over age 80 have it. With the increased numbers of people aging in the United States, more people are likely to have the condition in the future. In elderly people, it is associated with a higher mortality rate and more complications than in younger age groups. In this chapter, we look at the special conditions and needs in elderly people with heart failure.

AGING ARTERIES

As we grow older, we can feel our ligaments and joints stiffening. Walking gets harder. Even getting up from a chair takes more time. Knees may start to hurt. Although we can't feel it, our heart and arteries also stiffen with age. What we do sense, as a result, is that our exercise capacity decreases, and we find that we just cannot do the things we once could. In elderly people who develop heart failure, the stiffening of the heart and arteries is accelerated.

In healthy young and middle-aged people, major arteries, particularly the aorta, are flexible. With each contraction of the heart, blood is ejected into the arteries, which expand slightly to accept the blood. As the arteries expand, they absorb some of the increased blood pressure—some of the pressure is used up expanding the walls.

But in an elderly person whose arteries have stiffened, the heart is ejecting blood into a tube that resembles a copper pipe. The stiffer pipe doesn't expand, and therefore the blood pressure experiences the full effect of the bolus of blood entering the arteries. Accordingly, the person's blood pressure is elevated, particularly the systolic blood pressure. High blood pressure, in turn, means that the heart is carrying an extra load, because with every beat the heart must work to overcome the pressure. As the heart works harder, walls of the heart's left ventricle will thicken, or *hypertrophy*. The hypertrophy then leads to a stiffening of the heart, which makes it harder for the left ventricle to fill adequately. That is why in elderly people, often the left ventricle ejects blood normally but does not fill particularly well. If this process continues or accelerates, it leads to heart failure.

Elderly people often have many other diseases that worsen heart failure and complicate diagnosis and treatment. Coronary artery disease, diabetes mellitus, kidney problems, obstructive pulmonary disease, to name but a few, are all more common in elderly people. Some older people develop a degree of cognitive impairment that complicates compliance with a difficult medical regimen. Social issues such as the expense of medications not covered by insurance are a major reason elderly people have a higher mortality rate and tend to have more hospital admissions for heart failure than younger people with the same condition.

People who are 80 and older who have heart failure are treated with the same medications as similar but younger patients and respond to ACE inhibitors and beta blockers as well as younger individuals do. Doses need to be adjusted, though, because of the decreased muscle mass and mild kidney dysfunction common in elderly people.

MULTIPLE MEDICATIONS

Multiple medications are a big concern in older people. As we age, our ability to eliminate certain drugs becomes impaired. This leads to drug interactions not commonly experienced by younger people. Almost any drug may have unwanted consequences in elderly people. Be sure to speak with your doctor about drug side effects. Ask if what you experience as unwanted is commonly seen or is unique to you. Ask if there are other drugs you might try instead.

The other issue with multiple medications is remembering to take them. No pill will help you if it remains in the jar. Organization is key. Keep a list of your medications and update it religiously. Lay out your medicines in a pill sorter one week at a time. Do not allow your medications to run out without getting a refill. It is difficult to take multiple medications different times of the day. Use all the help you can get from your family and pharmacy.

Go over your medications each and every time you see your doctor. Remember that each medication has a trade name and a generic name. You do not want to be taking the generic metoprolol succinate and the trade name Toprol XL at the same time, for example. This would double the amount of this medication you are taking. If you have any doubts or concerns, ask your pharmacist or your doctor for help. Pharmacies may be able to place your weekly pill regimen in daily dosage containers for you. And visiting aides or nurses can come to your home to help you take your pills correctly.

LIFE CHOICES

Physicians try to relieve symptoms and prolong life. Once people are in their eighties, the majority of their life is behind them. As a patient, if you are very sick and medications or devices are not helping you have a good quality of life, you might decide that prolonging life is no longer your goal. Perhaps you do not want to tolerate side effects from drugs or devices that prolong life if they do not also improve your quality of life. Perhaps you are willing to trade quantity for quality of life. This is a personal decision and can, of course, be a decision made at any age. You must let your doctor know your goals. If he does not bring up the topic, you should.

Your doctor should be willing to listen to your concerns and help set up end-of-life care, perhaps even through a hospice program. Make sure that your doctors and your family all know your wishes. Many families struggle to make this decision for a loved one who was unwilling to discuss the issue prior to becoming unable to do so. I (Ed) have seen the hurt and turmoil this can cause. Do not let this happen to your loved ones. Have a plan and make your plan clear to all those who might be asked to make a decision about your wishes. Do not speak with only one of your children and assume she will speak with the rest. Speak to all of them. Make your wishes clear in a written living will or a health care power of attorney as well. If you become unable to communicate your wishes about your own care, a living will that you previously wrote will instruct your medical caregivers and your family on whether to use life-prolonging measures and in what circumstances you would not want such life-prolonging measures as being placed on an artificial respirator that breathes for you or being fed by a tube into your stomach if you are unable to eat. Be specific in listing what treatment you would and would not want under what circumstances. Get advice about how to write this from your doctor, lawyer, and family. But then be sure that it is only your wishes that you write down. A health care power of attorney designates a specific person to make these decisions for you in the event you are not able to communicate your wishes yourself.

I have many elderly patients, and most of them find that the impact of the normal cardiovascular changes associated with aging on their quality of life is modest rather than life altering or severely limiting. Many of my patients over age 80 with heart failure enjoy their lives. The condition is common in elderly people, but you should not believe that it is inevitable. If you have heart failure and are elderly, you must be organized or get help to be organized. Discussing your goals with both your doctor and your family is important and will help you live the kind of life you want to live. I assure you that heart failure need not prevent you from enjoying life at any age.

17

What You Can Do for Yourself

GET AN ATTITUDE

Did you ever play a sport? Think back to fielding a ground ball in baseball, or taking a free throw in basketball, or standing over a putt in golf. If the thought went through your mind that you might let that ground ball go through your legs, or miss that free throw, or leave that putt a foot short—you probably did. Attitude is part of the attack plan in sports. It is embedded in who an athlete is. Athletes at the top of their game have a swagger. Think of Ray Lewis, Mia Hamm, Derek Jeter, Lance Armstrong. You've seen them project a confidence that they will get the job done. Their confidence comes from their hard work, practice, talent, focus, discipline, intent to win, and a special effort they manage to give, especially in a clutch situation.

We want you to develop a swagger about living well with heart failure. Just as you knew you could scoop up that ground ball and start a double play, believe you will deal with heart failure and be successful. But having such confidence without doing the work needed to be able to field a ground ball is foolhardy. In sports, confidence comes from conditioning your body, knowing how to play the game, and practice—so much practice that you will rarely get it wrong. In heart failure, the confidence also comes from taking care of your body, knowledge, and practice: knowledge about your own particular heart failure and how to treat it and keep it at bay, and practicing everyday habits that will help protect your heart.

PUT YOUR HEART FAILURE FIRST

When you first develop the symptoms of heart failure and then learn from a doctor that you have it is the time to be preoccupied with yourself—how you feel and what choices you will make to get better. Focusing on yourself and your heart failure during this time is not at all selfish. It's smart and is your first step to regaining your health. During this time when you are seeing doctors and may even be hospitalized, you are, first of all, a patient. The rest of your life is pretty much on hold, and that's as it should be.

THEN PUT YOUR HEART FAILURE IN ITS PLACE

Once you've had the tests you need, learned what is wrong with your heart, done the research to understand your problem and the choices you have, asked your doctors detailed questions, and believe you are on the right treatments to get better—then is the time to ease back into your normal life and begin to put heart failure in the background. I (Mary) remember telling Ed, at our second visit, that the difference between our last visit and this one was that "When you saw me before, I was a patient, and now I'm a human being." What I meant was that the first time I saw him I was totally taken up with the state of my health and what I could do to keep from getting worse and even get better. I had been in that state of being a patient for months since first getting diagnosed and searching for treatment. Two weeks later, I was no longer so worried, had moved past being a patient, and was fully absorbed in my work teaching writing at a university, co-editing a book, and working on the house I had recently bought. That's not to say you forget you have heart failure. You just put it in its place.

Attitude is first of all how you feel inside about living with a diagnosis of heart failure and developing with your doctor your own personal plan to conquer it. Then it is how you project yourself to others: family, friends, colleagues or co-workers—all the people you come in contact with through your work and in your personal life. If you relegate heart failure to the background, so will they. Be absorbed with something—your job, a pastime, grandchildren, pets, spouse, a very good friend, or someone you may not know so well yet but who really needs your attention and help.

Through the bad times and the better ones, keep a sense of humor. Find something to laugh about every day. Enjoy living. Do things that are fun. And get plenty of sleep. See if you don't feel better if you're in bed by 10 at night. Don't wait until you're feeling overtired to go to bed. Then it's all the harder to get to sleep. My mother, a registered nurse, used to tell me that, and it's one of those wise things mothers say that are true. Having a good night's sleep is the best way to start the next morning with a great attitude.

TAKING CARE OF BUSINESS

Too often what we wish we would do and what we actually do are not the same thing. That darn free will we have gets in the way. Those of us who have been told we have heart failure know it is a serious diagnosis, and we have to get serious in our commitment to do what we are supposed to do each day to take care of our hearts. Look at it as taking care of business, doing what you have to do to get the job done. Some things we need to do are easier than others. Taking your medications correctly is one of the easier things you will need to do.

Medications

Learn what your medications do for you and take them faithfully every day. Get your prescriptions refilled before you run out. Be aware of possible side effects, and speak to your doctor if you think you have developed one. Remember that side effects may not begin until months after you have been taking a new medicine. Keep an updated list of your medications, including name, strength, and number of times per day you take each medicine.

If you take a lot of medications every day at different times of the day, develop a system for keeping track of what you take. Pauline (Peggy) Sloan, a Maryland woman in her eighties who lives at home and prides herself on being well organized, takes lots of different medicines every day and doesn't want to worry about taking the caps off her pill bottles each time. So she does it only once a month and puts all the pills she takes for one day into a plastic sandwich bag, filling 30 or 31 sandwich bags with a day's worth of all her different medications. Then each morning she takes one sandwich bag of pills and sorts them into the ones she takes in the morning, midday, and evening.

If you have only a few pills to take, you may want to write down what you take and the time you take it. But the moment you plop the pill in your mouth, have a pen in hand to mark down what you took. It's really easy to forget whether you have taken a certain medication if you don't have a way of keeping track of what you took. I have had it happen that I am holding a bottle of medicine in my hand and get distracted by something—someone calls or my little orange "monster" cat, who has no social skills, jumps on another cat, who screams. When the interruption is over, I look down at the medicine bottle and can't remember whether I took the pill or not. That's a good reason to use the pill-sorting method so that if you have laid out only that one day's supply of medicines in a pill tray or plastic bag and the pill is still there, you know you haven't taken it. If you're holding an entire bottle of pills in your hand, there is no way to know for sure whether you took that day's medicine or not. Not remembering if you took your medicine is not a sign of senility. When you do the same thing day after day, or if you are someone who has to take medicine three times a day, it simply is hard to remember if you just took a pill or if you're remembering taking a pill yesterday or this morning.

Find a way that works for you to be sure you take your medicines faithfully. If you need help, call on a family member or neighbor or get a visiting nurse or aide to come to your home. And if you don't know whether you took that day's medicine or not, err on the side of caution. Don't take it. Wait till the next day at the regular time to take the medication. Better to skip one day than to take a double dose.

Record your weight daily, dressed the same way, on the same scale, and at the same time of day. Unless you have consumed lots more calories than usual for a few days, rapid weight gain indicates fluid retention and precedes congestion. Press on your ankles with your thumb to see if you leave an indention. That is another sign of fluid retention and signals the need to take a diuretic or to increase the dose if you are already on one. Understand how to adjust your diuretics based on your daily weight. Discuss this with your doctor before changing your own medication habits.

Avoid medications that cause you to retain fluid. The most common over-the-counter culprits are the nonsteroidal anti-inflammatory drugs such as ibuprofen. There are others as well. Use acetaminophen to treat pain. Avoid most herbal remedies that you have not discussed with your doctor. Herbal remedies may help, but they can also hurt. Just because something is "natural" does not necessarily mean that it is safe. It may not be safe in the setting of heart failure. Of course, never use illicit drugs such as cocaine.

Diet

If your doctor has told you to restrict fluids, watch how much you drink every day. If you want to relieve congestion, you need to excrete more water than you drink. Johns Hopkins nurse practitioner Gail Hefter tells patients that if you have active heart failure, all fluids you consume in a day should fit into one two-liter bottle. Drinking more than that makes the heart work harder.

If you are an alcoholic, don't take a drink. If you are not an alcoholic but drinking alcohol is what caused the cardiomyopathy that brought on your heart failure, don't take a drink. If you have active heart failure, an alcoholic drink or two a month is more than enough. If you have gotten over your heart failure, a drink a day is okay, and some studies have found that it is actually good for your heart.

Do not eat a high-salt meal. That can be one of the harder things to do for yourself, because so many foods we eat in the United States are loaded with salt. Read labels and know the sodium content of food before you eat it. Keep chapter 12 by nutritionist Samantha Heller handy where you can refer to it, and make use of those fast food Web sites she recommends so that you know what's okay to eat and what's definitely not okay before you drive through a fast food restaurant again. Limiting your sodium is very important to help avoid fluid retention.

Avoid trans fats in the foods you eat. Trans fats are the worst fats. Be a label reader. If a food you start to buy says anything other than 0 g (grams) beside the words "trans fat," put it back on the shelf. Don't compromise on that. When you buy baked goods from a bakery counter, ask if the chef makes anything with trans fats. Better yet, make your own desserts.

Flax-Flips

Here's a quick and tasty dessert from a Johns Hopkins cardiologist, Sheldon H. Gottlieb, whose complete diet, *Greens, Beans, and Leans,* can be found at www.greensbeansandleans.com:

1. **Beat two egg whites till firm (use a small whisk).**
2. **Add a heaping tablespoon crushed flax meal and beat with whisk.**
3. **Fry on griddle in olive or canola oil.**

Makes three 2-inch flax-flips, which freeze well and defrost quickly in the microwave. Serve with low-sugar syrup and crushed fresh strawberries.

Daily Living

If you spend most of your time at home, either because you work from home or because you are no longer working, it is very easy to find yourself sitting most of every day. Be on guard, knowing that your body needs to stay active. You can do marching exercises seated in your chair. Or stand up and hold on to the top of an upholstered chair or some other object that won't move and march in place. Get up and walk around every so often. Exercise. Keep your legs and arms and the core of your body strong by following an exercise program that's appropriate for you. Exercise will tone your muscles and help you feel better and stay more independent. Do your stretching exercises every day, walk or ride your bike five to seven times a week, and, if you are healthy enough, do resistance exercises three times a week. When you exercise, you take charge of your body and your heart failure. This helps you not only physically, but psychologically. Hey, who's in charge here? I am.

Do not smoke. No compromise on that. If you do not smoke, don't take it up. If you do smoke, stop.

If you want to find a way to know other people who share your diagnosis, offer to start a support group at your local hospital. You can shape it into whatever you and others in the group want it to be. Bring in speakers on nutrition, new treatments, how to handle depression. An exercise specialist can lead your group in exercises you can do at home.

You may have spinoff groups of people who enjoy reading books and form a book club, or meet for group exercise with the exercise specialist, or form a cooking club with the challenge of creating tasty recipes made with no salt and no or little bad fats. Those who use computers may enjoy exchanging e-mail addresses and keeping in touch between group meetings through e-mail and social media such as Twitter and Facebook.

Depression makes heart failure worse and increases the risk of dying. The research is very clear on this issue. Signs of depression include a lack of enjoyment of life, difficulty sleeping, feelings of uselessness, poor appetite, and social avoidance. If you feel depressed, discuss this with your doctor. You may need treatment. There are medications that relieve depression and do not worsen your heart failure. Depression is a disease and not a moral problem. It is not something you can beat by simply saying you will adopt a more positive attitude. Take care of yourself. Please get help if you need it.

HELP SOMEONE

We all go through periods with heart failure when we need help. During these times, we're focused on trying to get better. If we're fortunate, others help us. When we do get better, it can be our turn to reach out and help someone. You'll find more than one way. You may start doing more around the house, helping ease the workload of those you live with. You may focus on being a friend to someone. You could volunteer as a tutor to help a child learn to read or catch up in school, or get involved in a program that feeds hungry children or homeless people. You may start that support group for people with heart failure or help out at your place of worship. Your local animal shelter has a pet who desperately needs a loving home. All you have to do is think about it and you'll find a way to be a buddy.

18

Where to Find More Information

One reason we decided to write this book is that the Internet has many outdated concepts and old facts about heart failure that are unnecessarily frightening. Yet we know, of course, that many aspects of heart failure will change in the years to come, and you will want to keep up with these new findings. We plan to update this book periodically, but the news and the Internet will provide updates more quickly than a book can do. Therefore, as you search for information, learn to choose Web sites and medical journals wisely, and even then be prepared to filter out old data about heart failure.

THE WEB

In this day of information overload, finding more information is not usually the problem. If you go to any of the Internet search engines, such as Google or Yahoo, you will find millions of Web site references to heart failure and more than a million for arrhythmia, heart transplant, and sudden cardiac death. The issue is not finding information; the issue is finding reliable information.

Here are the basic points to keep in mind about health care Web sites: many have another agenda. Web sites hosted or written by pharmaceutical companies or device companies want to sell their product. Universities, hospitals, and physician groups want to sell their services. Professional societies have Web sites aimed toward their members, though some have sections especially for the public. It is not that solid, reliable information cannot be obtained from any such Web sites; rather, you have to review these sites with their other agenda in the forefront of your mind. Be especially cautious when visiting Web sites that use ads or send ads to your e-mail address or that do not declare who is sponsoring the Web site and managing its content. A physician sending messages to your e-mail address trying to sell you products is very unusual conduct. It is wise to check with your own doctor and the Web site of the U.S. Food and Drug Administration (FDA) before spending money on a product that a doctor or anyone else tries to convince you to buy, especially if that doctor or other person makes money from selling you the product.

Some Web site addresses may change. If you don't find one you are looking for, put the name of the organization or group that runs it into a search engine to locate the current Web site.

Recommended Web Sites

The heart failure page on Medline Plus, at www.nlm.nih.gov/medlineplus/heartfailure.html, sponsored by the U.S. National Library of Medicine and the National Institutes of Health, is a great place to start. This site has patient education videos and multiple links with pages available in Spanish; it is very useful not only for heart failure, but for just about any medical problem. From Medline Plus you can click on "Other Resources" at the top of the page to go to the MEDLINE/PubMed Web site at www.ncbi.nlm.nih.gov/pubmed. This site provides access to many medical and scientific journals.

The American Heart Association at www.americanheart.org offers education and tips about living with heart failure and, as you would imagine, about all kinds of heart matters, including cholesterol, coronary artery disease, and much more. Check out their "Heart and Stroke Encyclopedia." You may want to make use of "Heart Profilers," which tells you about different treatment options for your heart problem (go to www.hearthub.org, then click on "Treatment Options" at the bottom of the page).

The Heart Failure Society of America has a number of excellent patient education modules about heart failure at www.abouthf.org. We especially appreciate that both the Heart Failure Society of America and the American Heart Association are more upbeat about living with heart failure than many other sites you may find on the Internet.

The Cochrane Collaboration: Cochrane Reviews Web site, at www

.cochrane.org/reviews, contains review abstracts and some plain language summaries of journal studies. The reviews discuss evidence for and against the effectiveness of treatments for all kinds of health problems. The Cochrane Library publishes complete reviews four times a year. The Cochrane Collaboration is an international independent and nonprofit organization with an excellent reputation.

There are also very useful Web sites sponsored by either individuals or small associations. One, CHFpatients.com, operated by Jon, who says he was diagnosed with congestive heart failure (CHF) some time ago, bears the logo "For CHF patients. By CHF patients." This site is an engaging, easy-to-read resource that covers almost any aspect of heart failure you would be interested in. There is also an area where people with heart failure can exchange ideas and experiences.

The Hypertrophic Cardiomyopathy Association has a very useful Web site with several important links at www.4hcm.org.

The Heart Rhythm Society Web site, at www.hrspatients.org, has information about the diagnosis and treatment of arrhythmias. The patient information page has links to many heart rhythm disorders, including long QT syndrome.

Manufacturer Web sites provide information about how pacemakers, implantable cardioverter defibrillators, and assist devices look and how they work. Put the name of the manufacturer into a search engine to find relevant sites.

How to Get E-Mail Alerts on Heart Failure

You can sign up for e-mail alerts to news about heart failure from a search engine such as Google News Alerts. But be prepared to get daily alerts and understand that what plops into your inbox will range from articles written about drug treatments for heart failure and news about genetics and heart failure to a story about someone in the news dying of heart failure.

You can learn of new medical journal articles on heart failure and related topics by signing up for free alerts with the journal *Circulation* at their Web site http://circ.ahajournals.org/cgi/alerts or by registering with PubMed. See www.nlm.nih.gov/bsd/disted/pubmed.html for tutorials on using the site, including a short tutorial on saving searches and getting updated searches e-mailed to you.

MEDICAL JOURNALS

Articles in medical journals are not written with the public in mind, although there are exceptions. The *Journal of the American Medical Association* has what it calls "Patient Pages." For the most part, however, what you will find is written in scientific jargon for doctors and other health professionals. These articles include reports on new research and new treatments, and meta-analysis reports by a doctor or scientist who has combed the medical literature and written a summary of what all articles on a certain topic have to say. Though these journals are not written for the public, you can learn to be a savvy consumer of journal articles on topics you educate yourself about. Essays and editorials are much easier to follow and understand than the research articles. Here are some tips for reading the medical literature.

The Most Reliable Journals

Not all journals are considered to be of the same prestige. The most carefully performed and interesting *clinical* research involving large studies conducted with patients to test a new drug, device, or other treatment, or a lifestyle change such as diet or exercise, will usually be published in one of the premier journals, such as the *Journal of the American Medical Association* (*JAMA*), the *New England Journal of Medicine* (*NEJM*), or *Lancet.* The leading cardiology journals are *Circulation* and the *Journal of the American College of Cardiology* (*JACC*). Major basic science articles are published in journals such as *Science* and *Nature. Nature* also publishes *Nature Medicine,* a journal of biomedical research. Articles published in these journals are peer reviewed, which means they are sent out to experts in the field to be scrutinized before they are accepted for publication, a measure intended to ensure accuracy and sound scientific reporting. The peer review system is an important guard for scientific publishing and for the protection of the public, but it is not foolproof. There have been occasions when data in a published article were later found to be made up or distorted, and the article was discounted. Journal editors have recently been discussing how to deal with conflict of interest by authors who write about a new treatment and who have financial ties to the company that manufactures the drug or device. This is a significant concern. Major journals require authors to list any potential conflicts of interest.

How to Read a Journal Article and Judge the Worth of a Study

Typically a journal article begins with an abstract that summarizes the study's findings. Read the "Background," "Methods," "Results," and "Conclusions." Then you might want to skip to the end of the article to read the "Discussion." If this article interests you, and if you are considering following through on the results of the study and trying to apply them to yourself, then go back and read the entire article, taking care to look for some of the following details.

Some studies are more important than others. The best clinical research is randomized, double blind, and placebo controlled or compared to an existing treatment, or both. These three criteria allow for the fairest test between two or more treatments or a new treatment and a placebo. Also, the more people involved in a study, the better.

Randomized means that people who participate in the study are assigned randomly to either the new drug being tested or to a drug currently available or a placebo. Randomization prevents researchers from "stacking the deck" by putting all the sickest patients in one group and the healthier patients in the other group.

A *placebo* is a pill that looks, smells, and tastes like the drug being tested but instead contains an inert ingredient.

Double blind means that neither the research participant nor the researcher knows which group the participant has been assigned to.

Size of the study matters because a study that includes thousands of people is more likely than a study of twenty people to represent what really happens in the population at large.

Major journals have a manuscript reviewed by an independent statistician before accepting it for publication. Look to see if the conclusions of the authors are justified by the data they present. Look at what controls the researchers used to guard against outcomes that could be the result of another condition, for example, or involve age or gender bias.

GUIDELINES FOR THE MANAGEMENT OF HEART FAILURE

Various organizations have prepared printed guidelines for the management of heart failure. The best of these are from the American College of Cardiology /American Heart Association, the Heart Failure Society of America, and the European Society of Cardiology. These guidelines can be found at their respective Web sites. Guidelines represent a combination of clinical research and expertise. They serve as the foundation for the diagnosis and care of patients. They are regularly kept up to date and are published in major cardiology journals. Unfortunately, they are not written for patients or their families but for a professional audience. Yet you will learn a good deal if you take the time to read them.

MEDICAL DICTIONARIES AND TEXTBOOKS

If you plan to read articles in medical journals and on Web sites and learn specific names for the human anatomy, you'll want to keep on hand a good medical dictionary, such as *Taber's Cyclopedic Medical Dictionary* or *Stedman's Medical Dictionary*. The American Heart Association has a "Cardiac Glossary" on its Web site (www.americanheart.org).

Medical textbooks are an excellent source for information but are written for medical professionals. The best starting point is one of the major cardiology textbooks, such as *Heart Disease,* edited by Eugene Braunwald, M.D. Such textbooks cover everything from the anatomy of the heart to the workings of the heart in health and disease, as well as treatments. *Gray's Anatomy* is a classic and can also be bought as an online edition. Your librarian will be able to direct you to other textbooks.

We highly recommend educating yourself about heart failure. The more you know, the better, we hope, you will live.

Epilogue

In the next decade, millions of people throughout the world will be told they have heart failure. That people will continue to get this disease is probably the most certain thing about it. Far less certain is the current state of treatment and prognosis. Outdated death statistics keep being published and recycled. These data do not reflect current and recent use of such life-altering treatments as beta blockers, ACE inhibitors, implantable cardiac defibrillators (ICDs), and heart transplants. A large, well-designed prospective study that enrolls thousands of patients of community physicians and academic medical centers is sorely needed to learn the true statistics for both overall death rates from heart failure and the rate of sudden death in people with heart failure. We propose that this study move forward as soon as possible. What a service it would be to patients, their families, and doctors alike to be able to see a true picture of heart failure in this century.

Another uncertainty we hope new research will help resolve is which patients will benefit from receiving an ICD. This is clearly a life-saving device for those at risk of sudden death who are otherwise in good health. The problem is in identifying exactly who those people are. Most people with heart failure and a low ejection fraction who get an ICD (who have not already survived an episode of sudden death) will not need the ICD, as evidenced by the fact that it never fires to correct a chaotic heart rhythm. Technological improvement also needs to be made to ensure that ICDs don't misfire when they are not needed, a painful and frightening experience for the person who wears one.

Finally, we wish that the medical community would come together and embrace a new name that better describes what is wrong with the heart. Getting this diagnosis is tough enough without hearing an inaccurate and needlessly scary name for it. Only a tiny minority of the hundreds of thousands of people who each year in the United States alone learn they have heart failure have a heart that has truly failed. The large majority have a condition that makes their heart unable either to fill properly or to pump properly, and that is a significant problem. But for many, it is a temporary problem. With the right treatment and what often seems like a little miracle to patients and caregivers alike, their heart regains normal or near normal power and ability to serve their body's needs.

Heart failure? No. Language failure, that's all.

We expect that the future for people told they have heart failure will continue to brighten if doctors will prescribe proven treatments outlined in national guidelines, and if those of us who get the diagnosis will take charge of our lives—eat diets low in sodium and saturated fats and free of trans fats, exercise regularly, and take our medications faithfully. A partnership between patients and their doctors based on knowledge, intent, trust, and persistence can build strong hearts.

And don't forget the swagger.

Appreciation

Thank you to every patient, named and unnamed, who shared your experience with us and gave us the benefit of your wisdom, grace, courage, and tips for living well with heart failure. We were so impressed with your cheerful outlooks and take-charge attitudes in helping yourselves get better and wanting to help others who have heart failure.

The work of many doctors, researchers, nurses, and others who care for people with heart failure is reflected in this book through the studies you led and participated in that found their way to medical journals, talks you gave in scientific meetings we attended at the American College of Cardiology, American Heart Association, and Heart Failure Society of America, and interviews and conversations we had with you. A special thanks to cardiology fellow Dr. James Mudd, who helped find research for some chapters of this book and is now a colleague on the faculty of the Johns Hopkins University School of Medicine. Thanks and kudos to nutritionist and friend Samantha (Sam) Heller, who wrote an excellent chapter on nutrition. Jacqueline Schaffer's outstanding illustrations help readers understand how their hearts work and some of the tests they may need to have. Copyeditor Melanie Mallon and senior production editor Courtney Bond made our book better by their careful attention to consistency and clarity.

I (Ed) thank my wife, Deborah (Debbi) Kasper, and my son, Edward (Ted) Kasper, for their patience, love, and understanding. I am pleased to say that none of Ted's lacrosse, basketball, or football games were missed during the writing of this book. I also thank my many colleagues at the Johns Hopkins Medical Institutions—a very special place indeed. I work with some of the premier cardiologists and cardiac surgeons in the world. They are a constant source of inspiration. One who inspired many of us through his loving care of his patients every day was my friend and mentor Kenneth L. Baughman, M.D., who tragically died in November 2009 and will be sorely missed. I am indebted to those I help train. By asking such thoughtful questions, the medical students, house officers, and cardiology fellows teach me far more than I teach them and keep me on my toes. A special thanks for the needed distraction provided by the Johns Hopkins University men's lacrosse and basketball teams. Go, Blue Jays!

I (Mary) thank special friends Dick Schaefer and Randy Rocha and my sister, Theresa Knudson, who look out for me in many ways. Appreciation also to two of the best writers in our field, friends Deborah Blum and Robin Marantz Henig, for discussing with me how to balance my personal experience with heart failure with the rest of this book. Buddy, Rudy, BB, and Sandy, who bore, not always patiently, the misery of my seeming to adopt a laptop as my favorite friend will soon get much more attention. Since saying that, I painfully lost my dear Buddy and BB, who did get much attention. For my welcome distraction, thank you, baseball! A special thanks to Yankees pitcher A. J. Burnett for sending me, by way of Randy, his signed baseball: "To Mary, Never give up!" Right back at you. Yankees, are you all fired up and ready to go to the World Series again?

May each of you in our extended family who experience heart failure keep your passions fired, whether in sports, music, reading, Twittering, gardening, family, pets, or whatever. Life gets too full of demands. We hope you find enjoyment and peace in every day.

Appendix

Trade Names and Generic Names of Drugs

This list of drugs is separated into categories by type of action. The drugs are listed in alphabetical order of trade name within each category. Not all of these drugs are used in heart failure. In fact, some of the drugs listed here may worsen heart failure. Many of the pills are combinations of two active drugs that fall under different categories. In this instance, the drug that belongs to the category under which the drug is listed is italicized. Some drugs are listed in more than one category. Chapter 5 provides details about the drugs commonly used in heart failure. The drugs marked with an asterisk (*) are approved by the Food and Drug Administration for the treatment of heart failure.

Trade Name	**Generic Name**
ANGIOTENSIN-CONVERTING ENZYME (ACE) INHIBITORS	
Accupril*	quinapril*
Accuretic	hydrochlorothiazide/*quinapril*
Aceon	perindopril
Altace*	ramipril*
Capoten*	captopril*
Capozide	hydrochlorothiazide/*captopril*
Lexxel	*enalapril*/felodipine
Lotensin	benazepril
Lotensin HCT	*benazepril*/hydrochlorothiazide
Lotrel	amlodipine/*benazepril*
Mavik	trandolapril
Monopril	fosinopril
Monopril-HCT	*fosinopril*/hydrochlorothiazide
Prinivil*	lisinopril*
Prinzide	*lisinopril*/hydrochlorothiazide
Tarka	*trandolapril*/verapamil
Uniretic	*moexipril*/hydrochlorothiazide
Univasc	moexipril
Vaseretic	*enalapril*/hydrochlorothiazide
Vasotec*	enalapril*
Zestoretic	hydrochlorothiazide/*lisinopril*
Zestril*	lisinopril*

Trade Name	**Generic Name**
ANGIOTENSIN RECEPTOR BLOCKERS	
Atacand	candesartan
Atacand HCT	*candesartan*/hydrochlorothiazide
Avalide	hydrochlorothiazide/*irbesartan*
Avapro	irbesartan
Benicar	olmesartan
Benicar HCT	hydrochlorothiazide/*olmesartan*
Cozaar	losartan
Diovan	valsartan
Diovan HCT	hydrochlorothiazide/*valsartan*
Hyzaar	hydrochlorothiazide/*losartan*
Micardis	telmisartan
Micardis HCT	*telmisartan*/hydrochlorothiazide
Tevetan	eprosartan
Tevetan HCT	*eprosartan*/hydrochlorothiazide
ANTIARRHYTHMIC AGENTS *Must be used with great care in heart failure*	
Betapace	sotalol
Cordarone	amiodarone
Mexitil	mexiletine
Norpace	disopyramide
Pacerone	amiodarone
Procanbid	procainamide
Pronestyl	procainamide
Rythmol	propafenone
Tambocor	flecainide
Tikosyn	dofetilide
BETA BLOCKERS	
Betapace	sotalol
Blocadren	timolol
Coreg*	carvedilol*
Corgard	nadolol
Corzide	bendroflumethiazide/*nadolol*
Inderal	propranolol
Kerlone	betaxolol

Trade Name	**Generic Name**
Levatol	penbutolol
Lopressor	metoprolol tartrate
Lopressor HCT	hydrochlorothiazide tartrate/ *metoprolol*
Sectral	acebutolol
Tenoretic	*atenolol*/chlorthalidone
Tenormin	atenolol
Timolide	hydrochlorothiazide/*timolol*
Toprol XL*	metoprolol succinate*
Trandate	labetalol
Visken	pindolol
Zebeta	bisoprolol
Ziac	*bisoprolol*/hydrochlorothiazide

CALCIUM CHANNEL BLOCKERS

Must be used with care in heart failure

Adalat	nifedipine
Caduet	*amlodipine*/atorvastatin
Calan	verapamil
Cardene	nicardipine
Cardiazem	diltiazem
Cartia XT	diltiazem
Covera HS	verapamil
Dilacor XR	diltiazem
Dilt CD	diltiazem
Diltia	diltiazem
Dynacirc	isradipine
Isoptin	verapamil
Lexxel	enalapril/*felodipine*
Lotrel	*amlodipine*/benazepril
Norvasc	amlodipine
Plendil	felodipine
Procardia	nifedipine
Sular	nisoldipine
Tarka	trandolapril/*verapamil*
Tiazac	diltiazem
Verelan	verapamil

Trade Name	**Generic Name**
CHOLESTEROL LOWERING	
Advicor	*niacin/lovastatin*
Altoprev	lovastatin
Antara	fenofibrate
Caduet	amlodipine/*atorvastatin*
Colestid	colestipol
Crestor	rosuvastatin
Lescol	fluvastatin
Lipitor	atorvastatin
Lofibra	fenofibrate
Lopid	gemfibrozil
Mevacor	lovastatin
Niaspan	niacin
Omacor	omega-3 fatty acids
Pravachol	pravastatin
Pravigard PAC	buffered aspirin/*pravastatin*
Questran	cholestyramine
Slo-niacin	niacin
Tricor	fenofibrate
Triglide	fenofibrate
Vytorin	*ezetimibe/simvastatin*
WelChol	colesevelam
Zetia	ezetimibe
Zocor	simvastatin
FORMS OF DIGOXIN	
Lanoxicaps*	digoxin capsules*
Lanoxin*	digoxin*
LOOP DIURETICS	
Bumex	bumetanide
Demadex	torsemide
Edecrin	ethacrynic acid
Lasix	furosemide

Trade Name	**Generic Name**
OTHER DIURETICS USED IN HEART FAILURE	
Often combined with a loop diuretic to increase urination	
Aldactone*	spironolactone*
Esidrix	hydrochlorothiazide
HydroDIURIL	hydrochlorothiazide
Zaroxolyn	metolazone
NITRATES	
Commonly used to treat angina	
BiDil*	hydralazine/*isosorbide dinitrate**
Dilatrate	isosorbide dinitrate
Imdur	isosorbide mononitrate
ISMO	isosorbide mononitrate
Isordil	isosorbide dinitrate
Monoket	isosorbide mononitrate
Nitro-Bid	nitroglycerin cream
Nitrodur	nitroglycerin patch
Nitrolingual	nitroglycerin spray
NitroQuick	nitroglycerin
Nitrostat	nitroglycerin
NONSTEROIDAL ANTI-INFLAMMATORY DRUGS (NSAIDS)	
People with heart failure should avoid these drugs or use them with great care and with permission of their doctor.	
Advil	ibuprofen
Aleve	naproxen sodium
Anaprox	naproxen sodium
Ansaid	flurbiprofen
Arthrotec	*diclofenac*/misoprostol
Bextra	valdecoxib
Cataflam	diclofenac
Celebrex	celecoxib
Clinoril	sulindac
Daypro	oxaprozin
Disalid	salsalate
Dolobid	difunisal
Feldene	piroxicam
Indocin	indomethacin

Trade Name	Generic Name
Lodine	etodolac
Mobic	meloxicam
Motrin	ibuprofen
Naprelan	naproxen sodium
Naprosyn	naproxen
Oruvail	ketoprofen
Ponstel	mefenamic acid
Prevacid Napra PAC	lansoprazole/*naproxen*
Relafen	nabumetone
Salflex	salsalate
Toradol	ketorolac
Vioxx	rofecoxib
Voltaren	diclofenac

OTHER DRUGS USED IN HEART FAILURE

BiDil*	hydralazine/isosorbide dinitrate*
Inspra	eplerenone
Natrecor*	nesiritide*

Notes on Sources

INTRODUCTION

Heart failure statistics come from this source:

Lloyd-Jones, D., et al. "Heart Disease and Stroke Statistics—2010 Update." A Report from the American Heart Association. *Circulation* 121 (2010): e1–e170. Published online before print December 17, 2009. A more recent version appeared January 26, 2010. http://circ.ahajournals.org/cgi/reprint/CIRCULATIONAHA.109.192667v1.

Most people with mild to moderate asthma can use a cardioselective beta blocker, such as metoprolol succinate, according to clinical studies, including those reviewed in this Cochrane report:

Salpeter, S., et al. "Cardioselective Beta-Blockers for Reversible Airway Disease." *Cochrane Database of Systematic Reviews,* no. 3 (2002). Art. No.: CD002992. DOI: 10.1002/14651858.CD002992. The Cochrane Collaboration is an international nonprofit organization that has a reputation for producing independent, carefully done systematic reviews of the effects of treatment, bad and good. The review cited looks at twenty-nine studies of patients with reversible airway disease (asthma or chronic obstructive pulmonary disease with a reversible obstructive component) and concludes that beta blockers that primarily work on the beta 1 receptor should not be withheld from heart failure patients with mild to moderate asthma. The authors noted that long-term use has not been established.

Communication with William Alvarez, pharmacist and clinical specialist in cardiology, Johns Hopkins Hospital: Of the three beta blockers used for treating heart failure, Alvarez says metoprolol succinate is the best because "it's more cardioselective. It hits the beta 1 receptor primarily." Co-author Mary Knudson has asthma, has used metoprolol succinate for five years, and has found that it does not block her ability to get relief from an asthma rescue inhaler, such as albuterol, when needed. Still, as Alvarez points out, doctors are cautious about giving a beta blocker to a person who has asthma, and each patient should be followed to be sure the beta blocker does not interfere with effective use of asthma medication.

CHAPTER 1. WHAT IS THIS THING CALLED HEART FAILURE?

The heart failure practice guidelines listed below provide a foundation for the diagnosis and care of patients with heart failure. They contain sections relevant to almost every chapter in our book. There is a great deal of agreement among the major guidelines. The stages of heart failure come from the American College of Cardiology Guidelines /American Heart Association. The definition of heart failure is common to all guidelines on heart failure.

Hunt, S. A., et al., American College of Cardiology /American Heart Association Task Force on Practice Guidelines (Writing Committee to Update the 2001 Guidelines for the Evaluation and Management of Heart Failure), "ACC /AHA 2005 Guideline Update for the Diagnosis and Management of Chronic Heart Failure in the Adult: A Report of the American College of Cardiology /American Heart Association Task Force on Practice Guidelines (Writing Committee to Update the 2001 Guidelines for the Evaluation and Management of Heart Failure)," *Journal of the American College of Cardiology* 20 (September 2005): e1–e82, and erratum in *Journal of the American College of Cardiology* 7 (April 2006): 1503–1505. The most recent update was made available April 2009. *Journal of the American College of Cardiology* 53 (April 2009): e1–e90. These guidelines of the American College of Cardiology and the American Heart Association cover adult chronic heart failure, including both heart failure with a weakened heart and heart failure with a normal ejection fraction.

Heart Failure Society of America, "Executive Summary: HFSA 2006 Comprehensive Heart Failure Practice Guideline," *Journal of Cardiac Failure* 12 (2006): 10–38. In addition to chronic heart failure in the adult, the Heart Failure Society of America Guidelines cover acute decompensated heart failure. This is another thoughtful and well-referenced guide for heart failure. It has a helpful section on what people with heart failure can do to help themselves.

Swedberg, K., et al. Task Force on the Diagnosis and Treatment of Chronic Heart Failure of the European Society of Cardiology. "Guidelines for the Diagnosis and Treatment of Chronic Heart Failure: Executive Summary (Update 2005): The Task Force for the Diagnosis and Treatment of Chronic Heart Failure of the European Society of Cardiology." *European Heart Journal* 26 (2005): 1115–1140. The drugs approved for use in Europe are slightly different than those approved for use in the United States of America. In addition to these European Society guidelines, there are also guidelines produced in Canada and Australia/New Zealand.

McMurray, J., and Swedberg, K. "Treatment of Chronic Heart Failure: A Comparison Between the Major Guidelines." *European Heart Journal* 27 (2006): 1773–1777.

CHAPTER 2. CORONARY ARTERY DISEASE

Lloyd-Jones, D., et al. "Heart Disease and Stroke Statistics—2010 Update." A Report from the American Heart Association. *Circulation* 121 (2010): e1–e170. Published online before print December 17, 2009. A more recent version appeared January 26, 2010. http://circ.ahajournals.org/cgi/reprint/CIRCULATIONAHA.109.192667v1. The statistics on coronary disease come from this reference. An abridged version of these statistics can also be found at the American Heart Association Web site: www.americanheart.org. These statistics are published annually.

Freeman, M. W., with Junge, C. *The Harvard Medical School Guide to Lowering Your Cholesterol*. New York: McGraw-Hill, 2005. The description of cholesterol in the first pages of chapter 2 comes primarily from pages 2–6 of this excellent book, which goes into more detail about cholesterol than you typically find in other discussions about cholesterol. Freeman and Junge make clear the less-known details about how cholesterol works in this understandable book for the lay reader.

National Heart Lung and Blood Institute, National Institutes of Health. *Detection, Evaluation, and Treatment of High Blood Cholesterol in Adults (Adult Treatment Panel III)*, 2002, updated in 2004. This is the guideline on cholesterol detection, evaluation, and treatment. It is the foundation on which all physicians should base their diagnosis and management of cholesterol as a risk factor in coronary artery disease. This is a detailed and dense report that deserves careful study. Table 2.1 comes from this guideline.

Dzau, V., et al. "The Cardiovascular Disease Continuum Validated: Clinical Evidence of Improved Patient Outcomes." Part 1, "Pathophysiology and Clinical Trial Evidence (Risk Factors Through Stable Coronary Artery Disease)." *Circulation* 114 (2006): 2850–2870.

Dzau, V., et al. "The Cardiovascular Disease Continuum Validated: Clinical Evidence of Improved Patient Outcomes." Part 2, "Clinical Trial Evidence (Acute Coronary Syndromes Through Renal Disease) and Future Directions." *Circulation* 114 (2006): 2871–2891.

The two articles by V. Dzau taken together provide a good understanding of cardiovascular disease as a continuum beginning with risk factors and ending with significant cardiovascular dysfunction. For those interested in the details, there is also an extensive reference list. Description of how a plaque develops, angina, and the development of myocardial infarction comes from these two articles.

Nabel, E. G. "Cardiovascular Disease." *New England Journal of Medicine* 349 (2003): 60–72. This article highlights what is known about genetic factors in cardiovascular disease. Several nice diagrams help explain cholesterol and metabolism. This is the reference for the information on risk factors for coronary disease found in this chapter.

The American Heart Association has excellent descriptions of high blood pressure and cholesterol problems on their Web site: www.americanheart.org. Spend some time navigating through the various pages, and you will find many interesting things.

Smith, S. C., et al. "ACC/AHA Guidelines for Secondary Prevention for Patients with Coronary and Other Atherosclerotic Vascular Disease: 2006 Update." *Journal of the American College of Cardiology* 47 (2006): 2130–2139. *Secondary prevention* is defined as the treatment of atherosclerotic disease after a cardiovascular complication such as a heart attack or stroke. This article is the reference for the treatment of risk factors after the development of myocardial infarction or angina. Ed and Mary agree that doctors need to be more aggressive about managing risk factors in patients who already have evidence of coronary disease.

CHAPTER 3. CARDIOMYOPATHY

Felker, G. M., et al. "Underlying Causes and Long-term Survival in Patients with Initially Unexplained Cardiomyopathy." *New England Journal of Medicine* 342 (2000): 1077–1084. This is a classic paper on the causes of dilated cardiomyopathy and is a source we used on that topic.

"Report of the 1995 World Health Organization/International Society and Federation of Cardiology Task Force on the Definition and Classification of Cardiomyopathies." *Circulation* 93 (1996): 841–842. We use this classification of the cardiomyopathies in our book.

"ACC/ESC Clinical Expert Consensus Document on Hypertrophic Cardiomyopathy: A Report of the American College of Cardiology Task Force on Clinical Expert Consensus Documents and the European Society of Cardiology Committee for Practice Guidelines." *Journal of the American College of Cardiology* 42 (2003): 1687–1713. Our information on hypertrophic cardiomyopathy draws from this outstanding document, covering all aspects of the disease.

Maron, B. J., and Salberg, L. *Hypertrophic Cardiomyopathy for Patients, Their Families and Interested Physicians*. 2nd ed. Malden, Mass.: Blackwell Publishing, 2006. This is an excellent book and must reading for all people with hypertrophic cardiomyopathy and their families.

Kushwaha, S. S., et al. "Restrictive Cardiomyopathy." *New England Journal of Medicine* 336 (1997): 267–276. This excellent description of restrictive cardiomyopathy is the source for our information on that topic in this chapter.

CHAPTER 4. DIAGNOSING HEART FAILURE AND ITS CAUSES

The best review is the ACC/AHA heart failure guidelines referenced in the sources for chapter 1. The other guidelines have good sections as well. While much of the information in this chapter about evaluating people with heart failure comes from co-author Ed Kasper's personal knowledge and experience, we drew on these guidelines in writing this section.

Hausleiter, J., et al. "Estimated Radiation Dose Associated with Cardiac CT Angiography." *JAMA* 301 (2009): 500–507. This study of 21 university hospitals and 29 community hospitals found that doses of radiation delivered in cardiac computed tomography (CT) angiography at the hospitals differed significantly. The study also showed that some effective ways to reduce radiation doses "are not frequently used."

Slørdal, L., and Spigset, O. "Heart Failure Induced by Non-Cardiac Drugs." *Drug Safety* 29 (2006): 567–586. A very complete review of noncardiac drugs that can precipitate or worsen heart failure symptoms.

CHAPTER 5. DRUG TREATMENTS

There are multiple guidelines for the management of heart failure in adults. In general, there is good agreement among the various guidelines. Some give greater weight to certain of the clinical trials than do others. In general, guidelines are written by groups of cardiologists expert in the management of patients with heart failure. The process is difficult and time consuming. A great effort is made to ensure that the guidelines are approved by other appropriate professional societies. Guidelines are designed for physician use and are not written with the lay audience in mind.

Hunt, S.A., et al., American College of Cardiology/American Heart Association Task Force on Practice Guidelines (Writing Committee to Update the 2001 Guidelines for the Evaluation and Management of Heart Failure), "ACC/AHA 2005 Guideline Update for the Diagnosis and Management of Chronic Heart Failure in the Adult: A Report of the American College of Cardiology/American Heart Association Task Force on Practice Guidelines (Writing Committee to Update the 2001 Guidelines for the Evaluation and Management of Heart Failure)," *Journal of the American College of Cardiology* 20 (September 2005): e1–e82, and erratum in *Journal of the American College of Cardiology* 7 (April 2006): 1503–1505. Updated April 2009 in *Journal of the American College of Cardiology* 53 (April 2009): e1–e90. All information on drug treatments can be found in this guideline.

Heart Failure Society of America. "Executive Summary: HFSA 2006 Comprehensive Heart Failure Practice Guideline." *Journal of Cardiac Failure* 12 (2006): 10–38.

Swedberg, K., et al. Task Force on the Diagnosis and Treatment of Chronic Heart Failure of the European Society of Cardiology. "Guidelines for the Diagnosis and Treatment of Chronic Heart Failure: Executive Summary (Update 2005): The Task Force for the Diagnosis and Treatment of Chronic Heart Failure of the European Society of Cardiology." *European Heart Journal* 26 (2005): 1115–1140.

ACE INHIBITORS

Multiple trials support the use of ACE inhibitors in heart failure. Below are three of the most influential clinical trials that have looked at this use, in patients with heart failure ranging from those who have asymptomatic left ventricle dysfunction to those with New York Heart Association Class IV heart failure.

The SOLVD Investigators. "The Effect of Enalapril on Mortality in the Development of Heart Failure in Asymptomatic Patients with Reduced Left Ventricular Ejection Fractions." *New England Journal of Medicine* 327 (1992): 685–691. This study established the benefit of ACE inhibition in a group of patients with asymptomatic reduced left ventricular ejection fraction. The benefit was in terms of the development of heart failure symptoms and a reduction in hospitalization as opposed to mortality. However, if this study is followed out far enough, it is likely that a reduction in mortality would also be found.

The SOLVD Investigators. "Effect of Enalapril on Survival in Patients with Reduced Left Ventricular Ejection Fractions and Congestive Heart Failure." *New England Journal of Medicine* 325 (1991): 293–302. This study looked at patients with a reduced ejection fraction and New York Heart Association Class II and III symptoms of heart failure. It established a mortality benefit to being on the ACE inhibitor enalapril as opposed to placebo. It is a classic study in the heart failure literature.

The CONSENSUS Trial Study Group. "Effects of Enalapril on Mortality in Severe Congestive Heart Failure: Results of the Cooperative North Scandinavian Enalapril Survival Study." *New England Journal of Medicine* 316 (1987): 1429–1435. This was the first of the ACE inhibitor trials to show a benefit in terms of mortality. Patients in this trial all had severe heart failure (New York Heart Association Class IV). It set the standard for ACE inhibitor trials to come.

BETA BLOCKERS

Carvedilol and metoprolol XL are the two beta blockers approved for use in heart failure by the FDA. What follows are some of the most influential trials of beta blockers in heart failure.

Packer, M., et al. "The Effect of Carvedilol on Morbidity and Mortality in Patients with Chronic Heart Failure." *New England Journal of Medicine* 334 (1996): 1349–1355. This was the first major trial of a beta blocker, in this case carvedilol, that showed a decrease in mortality. Patients in this trial all had an ejection fraction less than or equal to 35 percent. They were treated with digoxin, diuretics, and an ACE inhibitor. They were randomized to carvedilol versus placebo.

MERIT-HF Study Group. "Effect of Metoprolol CR/XL and Chronic Heart Failure. Metoprolol CR/XL Randomized Intervention Trial in Congestive Heart Failure (MERIT HF)." *Lancet* 353 (1999): 2001–2007. This is a nice example of a heart failure beta blocker trial that demonstrated a decrease in mortality in patients randomized to the beta blocker metoprolol CR/XL, also known as metoprolol succinate.

CIBIS-II Investigators and Committees. "The Cardiac Insufficiency Bisoprolol Study II (CIBIS-II): A Randomized Trial." *Lancet* 353 (1999): 9–13. Bisoprolol is a beta blocker widely used in Europe for the management of heart failure. The manufacturer of this drug has either not sought approval from the FDA or has not received it. In any case, the data are quite strong in support of bisoprolol also lowering mortality in patients with heart failure and a low ejection fraction.

Packer, M., et al. "Effect of Carvedilol on Survival and Severe Chronic Heart Failure." *New England Journal of Medicine* 344 (2001): 1651–1658. When beta blockers were initially being used in the management of heart failure, some physicians thought that beta blockers in patients with particularly severe heart failure would not be well tolerated because the drugs can worsen heart failure in this instance. This trial showed, however, that even patients with severe heart failure would tolerate and benefit from beta blockade.

The Beta Blocker Evaluation of Survival Trial Investigators. "A Trial of the Beta Blocker Bucindolol in Patients with Advanced Chronic Heart Failure." *New England Journal of Medicine* 344 (2001): 1659–1667. Unlike the ACE inhibitor trials, where virtually every ACE inhibitor studied showed a benefit in patients with heart failure and a poor ejection fraction, the same cannot be said of beta blockers. In this large study, the beta blocker bucindolol did not prove to be better than placebo in terms of probability of survival. The reasons for this are likely numerous. This could possibly be a drug-specific effect in that bucindolol simply doesn't work in heart failure. An alternative explanation is that the patients enrolled in the bucindolol study were different. Unlike clinical trials of other beta blockers, there was great effort made to enroll African Americans in the bucindolol trial. In any case, unraveling the answer to why bucindolol didn't work in heart failure will be very interesting.

LOOP DIURETICS

Numerous studies demonstrate the benefit of loop diuretics in the relief of congestion from heart failure and other disorders that cause congestion. There have been no randomized trials to date of loop diuretics and heart failure. This is because the relief of symptoms that loop diuretics provide is so pronounced that it would be unethical to randomize patients with significant heart failure to a loop diuretic versus placebo.

DIGOXIN

The Digitalis Investigation Group. "The Effect of Digoxin on Mortality and Morbidity on Patients with Heart Failure." *New England Journal of Medicine* 336 (1997): 525–533. This is the major trial that demonstrated that digoxin did not help people who used it live longer but did improve symptoms in 6,800 patients with heart failure who had symptoms. This is the reason why patients without symptoms of heart failure are not thought to benefit from digoxin. Because the drug does not prolong life, and patients without symptoms of heart failure cannot benefit from a reduction in symptoms of heart failure, digoxin is not used in asymptomatic patients with left ventricular dysfunction.

ANGIOTENSIN RECEPTOR BLOCKERS

There are several trials of angiotensin receptor blockers in patients with heart failure and a weakened heart muscle or reduced ejection fraction. A particularly good one is listed below.

Granger, C. B., et al. "Effects of Candesartan in Patients with Chronic Heart Failure and Reduced Left Ventricular Systolic Function Intolerant to Angiotensin-Converting Enzyme Inhibitors: The CHARM-Alternative Trial." *Lancet* 362 (2003): 772–776. This trial established the benefit of switching to an angiotensin receptor blocker if patients are intolerant of ACE inhibitors. The usual reason for this intolerance is a cough.

Yusuf, S., et al. "Effects of Candesartan in Patients with Chronic Heart Failure and Preserved Left Ventricular Ejection Fraction: The CHARM-Preserved Trial." *Lancet* 362 (2003): 77–81. There have been very few randomized trials of the management of patients with heart failure and preserved ejection fractions, the nonsystolic heart failure patient. This is the largest trial to date. Other trials are in progress. In this trial, patients with an ejection fraction greater than 45 percent and symptoms of heart failure were randomized to candesartan versus placebo. Those taking candesartan lived longer on average and had decreased symptoms. However, these differences were not statistically significant.

SPIRONOLACTONE

Pitt, B., et al. "The Effects of Spironolactone on Morbidity and Mortality in Patients with Severe Heart Failure." *New England Journal of Medicine* 341 (1999): 709–717. This was a large-scale and long-term study of low doses of spironolactone compared to placebo in patients with severe heart failure. There was a clear-cut reduction in risk of death. The investigators highlighted the importance of careful monitoring of kidney function and potassium levels.

ISOSORBIDE DINITRATE AND HYDRALAZINE

Taylor, A. L., et al. "Combination of Isosorbide Dinitrate and Hydralazine in Blacks with Heart Failure." *New England Journal of Medicine* 351 (2004): 2049–2057. This study looked at over 1,000 self-identified African Americans with heart failure and randomized them to a combination of isosorbide dinitrate and hydralazine or placebo. This trial showed that patients who took this combination drug in addition to ACE inhibitors and diuretics lived longer. It is uncertain whether Americans who do not self-identify as African American would also benefit from this combination because only African Americans were studied in this particular trial. The authors thought the combination drug would work well in African Americans based on previous research.

William Alvarez, pharmacist and clinical specialist in cardiology, Johns Hopkins Hospital, was a source for significant parts of the section on risks of drugs. In particular he pointed out the importance of getting all your drugs from one pharmacy so that the computer can check for drug interactions. He warned of the risk of heart attack if men take both nitrates and Viagra. His message is worth including, especially because he said that men frequently don't mention their erectile dysfunction to a doctor and just order Viagra from the Internet: "We've had several patients admitted to the CCU with a heart attack because they took their Viagra with their long-acting nitrate—because they both cause low blood pressure and vasodilation and cause your heart to increase its heart rate. If they're not taking nitrates, there's still a risk of heart attack if they take Viagra. Beta blockers are the biggest culprit in causing erectile dysfunction."

CHAPTER 6. CONVERSATIONS OF THE HEART

PACEMAKERS AND POSSIBLE WORSENING OF HEART FAILURE SYMPTOMS

Olshansky, B., et al. "Is Dual-Chamber Programming Inferior to Single-Chamber Programming in an Implantable Cardioverter-Defibrillator? Results of the INTRINSIC RV (Inhibition of Unnecessary RV Pacing with AVSH in ICDs) Study." *Circulation* 115 (2007): 9–16. This study addresses the issue of whether RV pacing the majority of the time is inferior to RV pacing only when needed and finds that it is not. This reference informs the part of chapter 6 that deals with the risks and benefits of standard pacing in patients with heart failure.

Wikoff, B. L., et al. "Dual-Chamber Pacing or Ventricular Backup Pacing in Patients with an Implantable Defibrillator: The Dual Chamber and VVI Implantable Defibrillator (DAVID) Trial." *Journal of the American Medical Association* 288 (2002): 3115–3123. This study suggests that right ventricular pacing is not good for patients with a weak heart. This is a smaller trial than the INTRINSIC RV trial listed above. Similarly, this reference deals with the risks and benefits of pacing in heart failure.

GUIDELINES

These are the references from which our information on pacing is largely developed. All three of the following practice guidelines reflect current management and are available at the American College of Cardiology Web site: www.acc.org.

Gregoratos, G., et al. "ACC / AHA / NASPE 2002 Guideline Update for Implantation of Cardiac Pacemakers and Antiarrhythmia Devices: Summary Article. A Report of the American College of Cardiology / American Heart Association Task Force on Practice Guidelines." *Circulation* 106 (2002): 2145–2161.

Fuster, V., et al. "ACC / AHA / ESC 2006 Guidelines for the Management of Patients with Atrial Fibrillation—Executive Summary: A Report of the American College of Cardiology/American Heart Association Task Force on Practice Guidelines and the European Society of Cardiology Committee for Practice Guidelines for the Management of Patients with Atrial Fibrillation." *Journal of the American College of Cardiology* 48 (2006): 854–906.

Blömstrom-Lundqvist, C., et al. "ACC/AHA/ESC Guidelines for the Management of Patients with Supraventricular Arrhythmias—Executive Summary: A Report of the American College of Cardiology/American Heart Association Task Force on Practice Guidelines and the European Society of Cardiology Committee for Practice Guidelines for the Management of Patients with Supraventricular Arrhythmias." *Journal of the American College of Cardiology* 42 (2003): 1493–1531.

BIVENTRICULAR PACING

Cleland, J. G. F., et al. "The Effect of Cardiac Resynchronization on Morbidity and Mortality in Heart Failure." *New England Journal of Medicine* 352 (2005): 1539–1549. In this classic study, 813 patients with severe heart failure, an ejection fraction of 35 percent or less, and left bundle branch block were randomized to conventional medical therapy or biventricular pacing (also known as cardiac resynchronization). They were followed for nearly 30 months. Biventricular pacing was shown to improve the symptoms of heart failure, increase the left ventricular ejection fraction, and decrease the risk of death.

Bristow, M. R., et al. "Cardiac-Resynchronization Therapy With or Without an Implantable Defibrillator in Advanced Heart Failure." *New England Journal of Medicine* 350 (2004): 2140–2150. This is another classic study of 1,520 patients with severe heart failure and left bundle branch block who were randomized to receive either optimal medical therapy alone or in combination with cardiac resynchronization therapy with either a biventricular pacemaker (no ICD) or a biventricular pacing defibrillator (ICD). Those in the study who got either device had fewer hospitalizations and lived longer than study participants who received only optimal medical therapy. Those who got a biventricular pacing defibrillator lived longer than those who got a biventricular pacemaker. This reference and the one previous to this speak to the risks and benefits of biventricular pacing and serve as the basis for much of what we say about that topic.

CHAPTER 7. STRAIGHT TALK ABOUT SUDDEN DEATH

Tomaselli, G. F., and Zipes, D. P. "What Causes Sudden Death in Heart Failure?" *Circulation Research* 95 (2004): 754–763. This is a very thoughtful article on the causes of rhythm disturbances leading to sudden death in patients with heart failure. This reference is a general source of data on the frequency, causes, and triggers of sudden death.

Sukhija, R., et al. "Implantable Cardioverter Defibrillators for the Prevention of Sudden Death." *Clinical Cardiology* 30 (2007): 3–8. An excellent review of the various trials that demonstrate the usefulness of defibrillator therapy in people with heart failure.

Greyson, B. "Dissociation in People Who Have Near-Death Experiences: Out of Their Bodies or Out of Their Minds?" *Lancet* 355 (2000): 460–463. Greyson has written an interesting account of the experiences reported by people who have survived a "near death" event. Our information on the near death experience largely comes from this reference.

GUIDELINES

Borggrefe, M., et al. "ACC / AHA / ESC 2006 Guidelines for Management of Patients with Ventricular Arrhythmias and the Prevention of Sudden Death—Executive Summary: A Report of the American College of Cardiology / American Heart Association Task Force and the European Society of Cardiology Committee Practice Guidelines." *Journal of the American College of Cardiology* 48 (2006): 1064–1108. This is another excellent practice guideline, giving a very detailed account of the current management of ventricular arrhythmias and prevention of sudden death. Many of the recommendations in this chapter on managing ventricular arrhythmias come from this source.

DEFIBRILLATORS IN CLINICAL PRACTICE

Tandri, H., et al. "Clinical Course and Long-term Follow-up of Patients Receiving Implantable Cardioverter-Defibrillators." *Heart Rhythm* 3 (2006): 762–768. This article followed 1,382 patients receiving an ICD from 1980 to 2003. It represents the use of ICDs at one institution, albeit the institution (Johns Hopkins) where the ICD was first used in a person. This source helps to define the risks and benefits of an ICD.

Cesario, D. A., and Dec, G. W. "Implantable Cardioverter-Defibrillator Therapy in Clinical Practice." *Journal of the American College of Cardiology* 47 (2006): 1507–1517. This is a well-written review article.

MAJOR CLINICAL TRIALS OF DEFIBRILLATORS

Bardy, G. H., et al. "Amiodarone or an Implantable Cardioverter-Defibrillator for Congestive Heart Failure." *New England Journal of Medicine* 352 (2005): 225–237. In this study, 2,521 patients with heart failure and an ejection fraction of 35 percent or less were all on standard heart failure therapy and were randomized to placebo, amiodarone, or a single-lead ICD. Amiodarone was no better than placebo. The study found after following study participants for five years that the relative risk reduction of death for ICD therapy compared to placebo was 23 percent and the absolute reduction of death compared to placebo was 7.2 percent. This is a classic publication and is sometimes referred to by its acronym SCD-HeFT. The reference to only 5 percent of patients with an ICD having an appropriate shock comes from this trial.

There are two points worth adding about this study:

1. An ICD does not prevent death from all causes, only from an abnormally rapid beat that causes the heart to shake and malfunction, such as ventricular tachycardia or ventricular fibrillation. Of patients wearing an ICD in this trial, 182 had died at the end of five years, compared to 244 in the placebo group.

2. This study tested the value of only one type of ICD, a single-lead ICD with specific programmed instructions on when to fire. The following paragraph from this study shows that patients considering ICD therapy should ask for some details from their doctor about what type of ICD they will get and what evidence there is that the type of ICD they would receive improves survival. Always ask if the risk quoted to you is the relative risk, which will be a much higher percentage because it compares the change in risk, or ratio, of the group that used a device or took a drug to that of a control group that did not use the device or drug, or the absolute risk, which is a subtraction of the lower risk caused by the device or drug from the control group. In this study, 29 percent of patients in the placebo group died, and 22 percent of patients in the ICD group died. Subtract 22 percent from 29 percent to get the actual, or absolute, reduction of death attributed to the ICD: 7 percent. So, for people involved in this study, their risk of dying improved by 7 percent. The study's authors made these important comments:

"It is critical to emphasize that the effect of ICD therapy in patients with CHF may differ substantially depending on the programming of the device; whether single-, dual-, or triple-chamber devices are used; whether antibradycardia pacing or rate-responsive pacing is used; which detection algorithm is used; and whether antitachycardia pacing maneuvers are used for ventricular tachycardia. Although physicians understand that different drugs lead to different outcomes, they may fail to realize that the same is true for ICD therapy. ICD therapy cannot be considered a single intervention, given the numerous possible permutations of this approach. Consequently, we cannot emphasize too strongly that we evaluated only very conservatively programmed ICDs with a conservative detection algorithm and shock-only therapy. We found strong evidence that this approach works; however, considerable caution should be used in extrapolating our results to other approaches to ICD therapy, such as those involving dual-chamber or biventricular pacing, since, as reported previously, they may not afford the same benefit or, for that matter, any benefit."

Moss, A. J., et al. "Prophylactic Implantation of a Defibrillator in Patients with Myocardial Infarction and Reduced Ejection Fraction." *New England Journal of Medicine* 346 (2002): 877–883. This is another classic paper that helped establish the effectiveness of ICD therapy. In this case, 1,232 patients with a prior heart attack and a left ventricular ejection fraction of 30 percent or less were randomly assigned to receive either an ICD or conventional medical therapy. During an average follow-up of 20 months, 19.8 percent of the patients died in the conventional therapy group, while 14.2 percent died in the ICD group. You may hear this study referred to as MADIT-II.

Shah, M., et al. "Molecular Basis of Arrhythmias." *Circulation* 112 (2005): 2517–2529. This is as good an explanation of the molecular basis of arrhythmias, particularly ventricular arrhythmias, as we could find. This was a source for the information on substrate for sudden death.

OTHER ARTICLES AND STUDIES ON DEFIBRILLATOR THERAPY

Stevenson, L. W. "Implantable Cardioverter-Defibrillators for Primary Prevention of Sudden Death in Heart Failure: Are There Enough Bangs for the Bucks?" *Circulation* 114 (2006): 101–103. This is a thoughtful article by a well-respected cardiologist pointing out that while ICDs save lives, medicine needs to do a much better job understanding who will actually need one. Much of the information on the question of who really needs an ICD comes from this source.

Desai, A. S., et al. "Implantable Defibrillators for the Prevention of Mortality in Patients with Nonischemic Cardiomyopathy." *Journal of the American Medical Association* 292 (2004): 2874–2879. This is an analysis of several different studies documenting that ICD therapy significantly reduces death in selected patients with heart failure due to a weakened heart muscle but no coronary disease. It had been argued that ICD therapy might not be as effective in those without coronary disease compared to those with coronary disease. This does not appear to be the case. This is the reference for the Dr. Desai quotation.

Teutenberg, J. J., et al. "Characteristics of Patients Who Die With Heart Failure and a Low Ejection Fraction in the New Millennium." *Journal of Cardiac Failure* 12 (2006): 47–53. This is a single center review from investigators at the Brigham and Women's Hospital, Harvard Medical School. They found that deaths occurred more frequently in patients with longstanding heart failure, repeated hospitalizations, severe symptoms, and kidney problems. Only 21 percent of deaths were sudden. This is the reference for the data presented in this chapter on the incidence of sudden death in advanced heart failure.

Lee, D. S., et al. "Effect of Cardiac and Noncardiac Conditions on Survival After Defibrillator Implantation." *Journal of the American College of Cardiology* 49 (2007): 2408–2415. In this study of 2,467 patients who received an ICD, investigators looked at why people died. They found that the sicker a patient was prior to ICD implant, the shorter his survival. This is not surprising. In this instance, and others like it in medicine, the more problems you have, the greater your risk of death. This study helps inform the question "who really needs an ICD?" as discussed in this chapter.

Hauptman, P. J. "Does It Matter Why and How Patients With Heart Failure Die? A Debate That Lives On." *Circulation: Heart Failure* 1 (2008): 89–90. In this editorial, Dr. Hauptman summarizes some of what has been learned from clinical trials studying death from heart failure, and he also points out difficulties and shortcomings inherent in such trials and in making comparisons between trials.

"We have in fact learned a great deal from a long list of studies: For example, patients with nonischemic cardiomyopathy can die of ischemic complications, implantable defibrillators may shift death from a sudden arrhythmic cause to progressive heart failure, and sudden death is clustered in the early period after myocardial infarction. Such analyses can also raise interesting hypotheses or help to demonstrate the robustness of a treatment effect, as, for example, when an intervention reduces both sudden and nonsudden causes of cardiovascular death. Many of these concepts apply not only to death as an end point but to any number of other cardiovascular events, such as stroke or nonfatal myocardial infarction.

"We also know that there are implicit limitations in all such studies, which are based in part on the lack of availability of comprehensive and relevant clinical data and on the definitions themselves. Long the purview of clinical trial events committees, these definitions may not be "user friendly" across clinical trials or be easily translated for use in large epidemiological databases. Even the simplest classification schema, such as arrhythmic death versus circulatory failure, can be criticized because of overlap and difficulties recreating the events that lead to death. Indeed, the fact that necropsy findings often do not correlate with "best estimates" from clinical data, including medical records, leads to even more uncertainty about whether we are really measuring what we think we are measuring. In addition, when it comes to categorizing a death, arguments can reach almost philosophical levels. What constitutes an arrhythmic death? Can a death be sudden if the patient has severe functional limitations and leads a New York Heart Association class IV existence? What does it mean if a drug or intervention causes a redistribution among the various causes of death without meaningfully affecting overall death rates?"

CHAPTER 8. SURGICAL TREATMENTS

Eagle, K. A., et al. "ACC/AHA 2004 Guideline Update for Coronary Artery Bypass Graft Surgery: Summary Article: A Report of the American College of Cardiology/American Heart Association Task Force on Practice Guidelines." *Circulation* 110 (2004): e340–e437. This practice guideline includes an excellent section on coronary bypass surgery in high-risk patients and in those with heart failure and is a source for information in this chapter on bypass surgery.

Jones, R. H., et al. "Coronary Artery Bypass Surgery with or without Surgical Ventricular Restoration." *New England Journal of Medicine* 360 (2009): 1705–1717. This article showed no difference in the combined incidence of death or hospitalizations between the group that received CABG versus CABG plus ventricular restoration.

Selzman, C. H., et al. "Surgical Therapy for Heart Failure." *Journal of the American College of Surgery* 203 (2006): 226–239. This is a thorough review of surgical therapy for heart failure, including heart transplantation, coronary artery bypass, aortic valve replacement, mitral valve repair, ventricular restoration, passive restraints, mechanical support, and the total artificial heart. Information on surgery for valve disease, passive restraint, and ventricular restoration comes from this source.

CHAPTER 9. DEVICE TREATMENTS FOR THE CRITICALLY ILL

See Selzman, C. H., et al., "Surgical Therapy for Heart Failure," in the previous chapter's sources. This article includes some informative photographs to help you understand what the total artificial heart looks like.

Gray, N. A., and Selzman, C. H. "Current Status of the Total Artificial Heart." *American Heart Journal* 152 (2006): 4–10. This is a complete review with some good photographs that show what the artificial heart looks like.

Miller, L. W., and Lietz, K. "Candidate Selection for Long-term Left Ventricular Assist Device Therapy for Refractory Heart Failure." *Journal of Heart and Lung Transplantation* 25 (2006): 756–759.

Rose, E. A., et al. "Long-term Mechanical Left Ventricular Assistance for End-Stage Heart Failure." *New England Journal of Medicine* 345 (2001): 1435–1443. This trial included 129 patients with severe heart failure who were not candidates for heart transplantation. The patients were randomly assigned either a left ventricular assist device (LVAD) or optimal medical management. At one year, survival in the LVAD group was 52 percent, and in the optimal medical group, 25 percent. However, at two years, survival in the LVAD group was only 23 percent, and in the optimal medical group it was 8 percent. It makes one wonder what we are actually doing using left ventricular assist devices in patients who are not candidates for heart transplantation because so few patients in either group survived two years. Are we only prolonging the inevitable? This is the source for the information on survival after LVAD or medical therapy noted in the chapter.

CHAPTER 10. GETTING A NEW HEART

Baumgartner, W. A., Reitz, B., Kasper, E., and Theodore, J., editors. *Heart and Lung Transplantation.* 2nd edition. Philadelphia: W. B. Saunders, 2002. This is the classic textbook on heart and lung transplantation. It includes excellent drawings. All the medical information about getting a heart transplant that is in this chapter can be found in this book.

Communication with John V. Conte, M.D., associate director of cardiac surgery and director, Heart Transplantation Program, Johns Hopkins Hospital.

The latest statistics on heart transplantation can be found at www.ustransplant.org.

MedlinePlus offers fair and unbiased information for the public at its Web site: www.nlm.nih.gov/medlineplus/hearttransplantation.html.

The International Society for Heart and Lung Transplantation Web site is for professionals, not patients: www.ishlt.org.

Another excellent textbook is

Kirklin, J. K., Young, J. B., McGiffin, D. C. *Heart Transplantation.* 2002. New York, Edinburgh, London, Philadelphia: Churchill Livingstone, Elsevier Science, 2002.

CHAPTER 11. FUTURE THERAPIES

Berenson, A., and Abelson, R. "The Evidence Gap: Weighing the Costs of a CT Scan's Look Inside the Heart." *The New York Times*, June 29, 2008. This is one source for cautioning consumers to bear in mind that owners of expensive CT scanners will pay for them by using them on patients.

Mudd, J. O., and Kass, D. A. "Reversing Chronic Remodeling in Heart Failure." *Expert Review of Cardiovascular Therapeutics* 5 (2007): 585–598. This is an outstanding review of chronic remodeling, the process by which the left ventricle goes from the normal football shape to a beach ball shape and how different therapies can reverse the remodeling and bring the heart back to its normal shape. It includes both pharmacological therapy and surgical therapy as well as genetic and cellular approaches.

Chen, S. Y., and Tang, W. H. W. "Emerging Drugs for Acute and Chronic Heart Failure: Current and Future Developments." *Expert Opinion in Emerging Drugs* 12 (2007): 750–795. This is a terrific review of new drugs for heart failure as of 2007. Most of the information on this topic comes from this review.

Konstam, M. A., et al. "Effects of Oral Tolvaptan in Patients Hospitalized for Worsening Heart Failure: The EVEREST Outcome Trial." *Journal of the American Medical Association* 297 (2007): 1319–1331. In this study of 4,133 patients hospitalized for heart failure, tolvaptan, a vasopressin antagonist, did not prevent patients from dying. Patients were randomized within 48 hours of admission to standard therapy or tolvaptan. While the drug did not extend life, it improved many of the symptoms of heart failure, and no adverse side effects were noted. This reference is mentioned in the chapter.

Mitrovic, V., et al. "Hemodynamic and Clinical Effects of Ularitide in Decompensated Heart Failure." *European Heart Journal* 27 (2006): 2823–2832. Ularitide is a drug much like B-type natriuretic peptide. This is a small study (221 patients) that shows beneficial effects in heart failure.

Costanzo, M. R., et al. "Ultrafiltration Versus Intravenous Diuretics for Patients Hospitalized for Acute Decompensated Heart Failure." *Journal of the American College of Cardiology* 49 (2007): 675–683. In this study, 200 patients were randomized to either ultrafiltration (removal of fluid similar to dialysis) or intravenous diuretics. Ultrafiltration produced greater fluid loss without any change in kidney function. This is the source for information about fluid removal found in this chapter.

Hagege, A. A., et al. "Skeletal Myoblast Transplantation in Ischemic Heart Failure: Longterm Follow-up of the First Phase I Cohort of Patients." *Circulation* 114 (2006): I-108–I-113. This is an example of the exciting field of cellular transplantation, in which cells taken from skeletal muscle, such as the thigh muscle, were injected into the heart muscle. It includes only nine patients but shows a steady improvement in ejection fraction. This is a source for the information on stem cells found in this chapter.

Jones, R. H., et al. "Coronary Artery Bypass Surgery with or without Surgical Ventricular Restoration." *New England Journal of Medicine* 360 (2009): 1705–1717. There does not appear to be a mortality benefit to surgical ventricular restoration when added to CABG.

Acker, M. A., et al. "Mitral Valve Surgery in Heart Failure: Insights from the ACORN Clinical Trial." *Journal of Thoracic and Cardiovascular Surgery* 132 (2006): 568–577. An interesting insight about mitral valve surgery and passive left ventricular restraints. This is a source we used for the information on passive restraints.

Burkhoff, D., et al. "A Randomized Multicenter Clinical Study to Evaluate the Safety and Efficacy of the TandemHeart Percutaneous Ventricular Assist Device Versus Conventional Therapy with Intraaortic Balloon Pumping for Treatment of Cardiogenic Shock." *American Heart Journal* 152 (2006): 469.e1–469.e8. The interesting idea here is that this is a ventricular assist device that can be placed into a patient in the cardiac catheterization lab and does not require a major heart operation and all the associated complications. This is the source used in our mention of assist devices.

Jourdain, P., et al. "Plasma Brain Natriuretic Peptide–Guided Therapy to Improve Outcome in Heart Failure." *Journal of the American College of Cardiology* 49 (2007): 1733–1739. This is a small study (220 patients with heart failure) that suggests that using plasma BNP levels can help guide therapy by increasing the dose of beta blockers and ACE inhibitors. This is interesting but not currently well accepted. The future of heart failure therapy may well include something like this—the use of biomarkers to guide therapy.

CHAPTER 12. NUTRITION AND HEART FAILURE

SODIUM AND POTASSIUM

USDA Center for Nutrition Policy and Promotion. *Insight 3: Dietary Guidance on Sodium: Should We Take It with a Grain of Salt?* Center for Nutrition Policy and Promotion, May 1997.

The USDA *Dietary Guidelines for Americans 2005* Web site, www.pyramid.gov, has much helpful information, including tips and resources, dietary guidelines, and information for kids. Many brochures are available as free PDF downloads. This is an excellent reference for data on sodium.

U.S. Department of Agriculture, Agricultural Research Service. *USDA National Nutrient Database for Standard Reference.* Release 18. www.nal.usda.gov/fnic/foodcomp/Data/SR18/sr18.html. If you want to know what is in a certain food, like frozen spinach, cereal, or a hamburger, you can go to the USDA Web site listed above. Click on "search" and enter the food you are interested in. You can get information on calories, fats, sodium, and other nutrients.

Jacobson, M. F., and Hurley, J. G. Center for Science in the Public Interest. *Restaurant Confidential.* New York: Workman Publishing, 2002. This book lists the nutrients in popular foods and in many restaurant foods. You will be stunned at the saturated fat and sodium in some of these foods. But the authors point out good choices, too.

FATTY ACIDS AND CHOLESTEROL

Willett, W. C., et al. "Intake of Trans Fatty Acids and Risk of Coronary Heart Disease among Women." *Lancet* 341 (1993): 581–585. The Nurses' Health Study began in 1976, when 121,700 U.S. female registered nurses completed questionnaires about their medical history. It is one of the largest ongoing prospective investigations into the risk factors for major chronic diseases in women. As such, studies continue to be reported from it.

Mozaffarian, D., et al. "Trans Fatty Acids and Cardiovascular Disease." *New England Journal of Medicine* 354 (2006): 1601–1613. Clinical studies are showing us that eating trans fats increases our risk for many chronic diseases. Studies in the *Lancet,* March 1993, and the *New England Journal of Medicine* in April 2006 are two notable examples. These and other studies provide the scientific basis that is causing lawmakers to urge removal of trans fats from foods, and many restaurants, fast food chains, and food companies to remove trans fats from their products.

Esposito, K., and Giugliano, D. "Diet and Inflammation: A Link to Metabolic and Cardiovascular Diseases." *European Heart Journal* 27 (2006): 15–20. This review describes the link between the fats we eat, inflammation, and cardiovascular and metabolic diseases.

The Harvard School of Public Health has a nice explanation of good and bad fats in its nutrition newsletter at www.hsph.harvard.edu/nutritionsource/fats.html.

American Heart Association. *Fat.* AHA Scientific Position. www.americanheart.org/presenter.jhtml?identifier=4582, 2005. This is the reference for how much saturated fat you can consume per day.

Albert, C. M., et al. "Blood Levels of Long-Chain n-3 Fatty Acids and the Risk of Sudden Death." *New England Journal of Medicine* 346 (2002):1113–1118. Omega-3 fatty acids may help prevent sudden death. Other studies support this statement.

SUPPLEMENTS

Zittermann, A., et al. "Low Vitamin D Status: A Contributing Factor in the Pathogenesis of Congestive Heart Failure?" *Journal of the American College of Cardiology* 41 (2003): 105–112. This study suggests that heart failure patients tend to be deficient in Vitamin D.

Hathcock, J. N., et al. "Risk Assessment for Vitamin D." *American Journal of Clinical Nutrition* 85 (2007): 6–18. These experts suggest that the upper tolerability limit for Vitamin D be raised to 10,000 IU.

Zittermann, A., et al. "Vitamin D Insufficiency in Congestive Heart Failure: Why and What to Do about It?" *Heart Failure Reviews* 11 (2006): 25–33. These researchers suggest that people with heart failure should take 50–100 mcg of Vitamin D daily.

National Institutes of Health. "Magnesium," Dietary Supplement Fact Sheet, updated July 13, 2009, http://ods.od.nih.gov/factsheets/cc/magn.html#what. Most Americans do not get enough magnesium in their diet.

Standing Committee on the Scientific Evaluation of Dietary Reference Intakes, Food and Nutrition Board, Institute of Medicine. *DRI: Dietary Reference Intakes for Calcium, Phosphorus, Magnesium, Vitamin D, and Fluoride.* Washington, D.C.: National Academies Press, 1997. This is the reference for the recommended daily oral intake for a variety of minerals, including calcium, phosphorous, magnesium, Vitamin D, and fluoride.

CHAPTER 13. EXERCISE

Many small studies show different benefits of exercise in people with heart failure. Some are tentative, and some are positive in showing benefit and no harm. Because so many individual studies are small, it is more helpful to look for review articles or meta-analysis articles. Two are cited below.

ExTraMATCH. "Exercise Training Meta-Analysis of Trials in Patients with Chronic Heart Failure." *British Medical Journal* 328 (2004): 189. BMJ online January16, 2004, 1–8. This meta-analysis found that exercise training significantly prolonged life and reduced admission to hospitals in patients with chronic heart failure due to left ventricular systolic dysfunction.

Stewart, K. J. "Cardiac Rehabilitation Following Percutaneous Revascularization, Heart Transplant, Heart Valve Surgery, and for Chronic Heart Failure." *CHEST* 123 (2003): 2104–2111.

HF-ACTION, by far the largest randomized exercise trial of people with heart failure, involving 2,331 patients from 82 medical centers, was reported on November 11, 2008, at the American Heart Association Scientific Sessions 2008 in New Orleans. The study, funded by the National Heart, Lung and Blood Institute, fell short of its hypothesis, which hoped to show that people with left ventricular systolic dysfunction who participate in a supervised exercise program involving bike riding or walking would have a 20 percent lower rate of hospitalization and of death from all causes at the end of two years. The small gains for the exercise group over the group that received optimal medical care but no exercise training were statistically insignificant. However, this large trial did demonstrate that exercise is safe for heart failure patients, and a substudy of the trial discussed on November 12 found that aerobic exercise improved patients' health.

Christopher O'Connor, M.D., of Duke University Medical Center, and David J. Whellan, M.D., of Jefferson Medical College, primary investigators of the HF-ACTION study, offered two reasons why the study may not have reached the primary endpoint the researchers had hoped for. Participants in the exercise arm of the study did not exercise as long and as often as the study called for, and participants in the usual care group did some exercising on their own, which could have diminished the results. Also, the best clinical studies are double blind, meaning that neither the patients nor their doctors know who is getting the tested treatment and who is getting the placebo or standard treatment. This is easy to do in a clinical trial involving a drug but was impossible to do in this trial, which involved exercise training for half the patients. Study participants had left ventricular systolic dysfunction, New York Heart Association Class II–IV symptoms, and an ejection fraction less than 35 percent; all were on optimal medical treatment and were capable of exercising. Slides and interviews with the study investigators can be found at directnews.americanheart.org.

CHAPTER 14. THE PATIENT-DOCTOR THERAPEUTIC RELATIONSHIP

These three books provide wonderful insights into doctor-patient relationships.

Callahan, D. *What Kind of Life.* New York: Simon and Schuster, 1990. This is an important book for anyone likely to come in contact with medicine and that is all of us.

Groopman, J. *How Doctors Think.* Boston: Houghton Mifflin, 2007. Dr. Groopman, chair of medicine at the Harvard Medical School, has an interesting take on how doctors think and why this might be important to you.

Reynolds, R., et al. *On Doctoring.* New York: Simon and Schuster, 2001. This beautiful collection of essays, poems, and stories written by a wide range of physicians and nonphysicians, including some famous writers, describes encounters of patients and doctors and their thoughts and feelings.

CHAPTER 15. WHAT YOU NEED TO KNOW ABOUT THE HOSPITAL

The following are references to the sections of this chapter that concern the risks of hospitalization.

Kohn, L. T., et al., editors. *To Err Is Human: Building a Safer Health System.* Washington, D.C.: National Academies Press, 2000. This is a thoughtful examination of medical error. It deserves careful reading.

Gawande, A. *Complications: A Surgeon's Notes on an Imperfect Science.* New York: Picador / Henry Holt, 2002. Atul Gawande is a surgeon at Brigham and Women's Hospital in Boston and a staff writer for the *New Yorker,* a first-rate journalist and a superb writer. His stories in *Complications* are entertaining as narratives and reveal truths about the complexities of being a doctor in a hospital setting. Gawande probes the uncertainties and unknowns involved in practicing medicine and describes the fallibilities of doctors. This book inspired Mary to develop a new course in training medical writers at Johns Hopkins University, and it is an important read for anyone wanting to understand in more depth and detail how doctors and hospitals work.

Gawande, A. *Better: A Surgeon's Notes on Performance.* New York: Metropolitan Books/Henry Holt, 2007. In his second book, Gawande continues his thoughtful and well-written pursuit of understanding the performance of doctors and what makes some better than others.

Brownlee, S. *Overtreated: Why Too Much Medicine Is Making Us Sicker and Poorer.* New York: Bloomsbury, 2007. Brownlee did a great deal of research to produce this book, which warns that much medical care has no scientific proof that it works and that hospitals can be dangerous places for many reasons, including a lack of coordinated care.

The following are references for the section on therapy in the hospital.

"Intravenous Nesiritide vs Nitroglycerin for Treatment of Decompensated Congestive Heart Failure: A Randomized Controlled Trial." *Journal of the American Medical Association* 287 (2002): 1531–1540. This study demonstrated the use of nesiritide (B-type natriuretic peptide) in the therapy of acute heart failure. Nesiritide relieved symptoms of acute heart failure, predominantly shortness of breath, more quickly than did a standard therapy for the condition—nitroglycerin. In stark contrast, the following study suggested that it may be associated with an increase in death risk. This is a controversial area and needs further research.

Sackner-Bernstein, J. D., et al. "Short-term Risk of Death After Treatment With Nesiritide for Decompensated Heart Failure: A Pooled Analysis of Randomized Controlled Trials." *Journal of the American Medical Association* 293 (2005): 1900–1905. This study set off a firestorm of controversy by suggesting that nesiritide increased the risk of death. This is a pooled analysis and not a randomized, controlled trial. It has been subject to much criticism. Most heart failure experts do not believe that nesiritide increases the risk of death. It has been shown to be effective when used to augment diuretics to decrease severe symptoms of volume overload.

Adams, K. F., et al. "Section 12: Evaluation and Management of Patients With Acute Decompensated Heart Failure. Heart Failure Society 2006 Comprehensive Heart Failure Practice Guideline." *Journal of Cardiac Failure* 12 (2006): e86–e103. The Heart Failure Society guidelines contain a particularly good section on the care of patients with heart failure in need of hospitalization.

Baughman, K., and Baumgartner, W. A. *Treatment of Advanced Heart Disease.* New York: Taylor and Francis, 2006. This is a very good book on the management of severe heart failure. There are excellent sections on drug therapy, device therapy, and surgical therapy.

CHAPTER 16. HEART FAILURE IN ELDERLY PEOPLE

The following are general references for the information found in this chapter. These are all thoughtful articles on heart failure in the elderly.

Kupari, M., et al. "Congestive Heart Failure in Old Age: Prevalence, Mechanisms and 4-year Prognosis in the Helsinki Aging Study." *Journal of Internal Medicine* 241 (1997): 387–394.

Krumholz, H. M., et al. "Readmission After Hospitalization for Congestive Heart Failure Among Medicare Beneficiaries." *Archives of Internal Medicine* 157 (1997): 99–104.

Doba, N., et al. "Drugs, Heart Failure and Quality of Life: What Are We Achieving? What Should We Be Trying to Achieve?" *Drugs and Aging* 14 (1999): 153–163.

CHAPTER 17. WHAT YOU CAN DO FOR YOURSELF

Adams, K. F., et al. "Section 6: Nonpharmacologic Management and Health Care Maintenance in Patients With Chronic Heart Failure. Heart Failure Society 2006 Comprehensive Heart Failure Practice Guideline." *Journal of Cardiac Failure* 12 (2006): e29–e33. Though not written for a lay audience, this is a good review of what you can do to help safeguard your health.

You can be a very good source for deciding what small and big things you can do in your daily life to get better from heart failure. You know what works for you. Take care of yourself.

Index